'In her gruesome book… Herman explores assassinations and stories of poison… and questions if some stories of death by poison could be inaccurate… truly scary.' *Daily Mail*, **Book of the Week (December 2018)**

'*The Royal Art of Poison* by Eleanor Herman will, for once in your life, make you happy you are not a princess or a queen or someone who lives in a palace. The book is amazing and really makes me wonder how we've managed to survive. It will make you glad to be in your own home.' *Forbes*, **'Books to Travel With for the Holidays'**

'An entertainingly gruesome journey through filth, poison and disease, pulsating with grim and entertaining anecdotes. Wickedly good.' **Longlisted for the 2019 HWA Non-Fiction Crown Award**

'Eleanor Herman provides an engaging and well researched account of the murky world of royal poisonings. Packed with interesting details, *The Royal Art of Poison* is a joy to read.' **Elizabeth Norton, historian and author of *The Hidden Lives of Tudor Women* and *England's Queens: The Biography***

'Rambunctious, rip-roaring history with the horrible bits left in, from medicines made from heavy metals or human flesh to poison preventatives and putrid palaces. But Herman's scouring of the records for cures that can kill also explains some real anomalies in the royal story.' **Sarah Gristwood, author of *Game of Queens: The Women Who Made Sixteenth Century Europe***

'Fascinating - and horrifying - in equal measure. Eleanor Herman draws the reader into a world in which the bizarre becomes normality, as she looks back through scandalous layers of history and reveals a deadly world of ubiquitous poisons.' **Lucinda Hawksley, author of *Bitten By Witch Fever***

'Herman shines the bright light of meticulous research into the murky underworlds of poison and politics. Deliberate, accidental, self-inflicted or medically prescribed, this is a treasure trove of surprises guaranteed to make your skin crawl. With delicious detail sure to turn your stomach, *The Royal Art of Poison* is a terrifying delight.' **Matthew Lewis, author of** *Survival of the Princes in the Tower: Murder, Mystery and Myth*

'Whether deliberate, accidental or the result of an antidote, the gruesome outcome of ingestion of toxins is deftly described in *The Royal Art of Poison*. Add political intrigue, disgusting sanitation, ubiquitous filth, horrendous medical procedures, and every sort of vermin and you get a very different picture to what we romantically assume to be the 'good old days.' **Penny Le Couteur, author of** *Napoleon's Button*

'Herman has a delightful appreciation for all things beautiful and terrible. With her dishy signature style and a dazzling command of the facts, she brews up a heady mix of erudite history and delicious gossip.' **Aja Raden,** *New York Times* **bestselling author of** *Stoned*

'A pernicious history that will make jaws drop and pages fly.' *Booklist*

'Rip-roaring pop history… by turns fascinating and stomach-churning, the book's detailed descriptions of different types of poisons will both shock and delight history buffs and enthusiasts of the macabre.' *Publishers Weekly*

'Luckily, we have *New York Times*-bestselling author Eleanor Herman to help us navigate an aspiring widow's bulging cabinet of nasty concoctions with her new book, *The Royal Art of Poison*. This fantastic work combines morbid curiosity and royal gossip. In it, readers will not only find out about who could've poisoned whom, but also why and with what. Lovers of Tudor history, costume dramas, and high fantasy will rejoice.' *Washington Independent Review of Books,* **50 Favourite Books of 2018**

the royal art of POISON

FATAL COSMETICS, DEADLY MEDICINES, AND MURDER MOST FOUL

ELEANOR HERMAN

DUCKWORTH

First published in the United Kingdom by Duckworth in 2019

Duckworth, an imprint of Prelude Books Ltd
13 Carrington Road, Richmond,
TW10 5AA, United Kingdom
www.duckworthbooks.co.uk
For bulk and special sales please contact
info@preludebooks.co.uk

A catalogue record for this book is available
from the British Library

Typeset by Jonathan Bennett

Printed and bound in Great Britain by Clays Ltd, Elcograf S.p.A.

ISBN 978-0-7156-5314-2

1 3 5 7 9 10 8 6 4 2

To Vladimir Kara-Murza, Russian activist and journalist,
who has survived Kremlin poisoning twice, living proof that
the royal art of poison did not die out with the Baroque
era but is alive and well in the digital age.

CONTENTS

Acknowledgments ix
Introduction xi

Part I Poison, Poison, Everywhere
1. Poison from the Banquet Table to the Royal Underpants 3
2. Unicorn Horns and Rooster Dung: Poison Detectors and Antidotes 19
3. Dying to Be Beautiful: Dangerous Cosmetics 31
4. Murderous Medicine: Mercury Enemas and Rat Turd Elixirs 43
5. Putrid Palaces: A Poisoned Environment 61

Part II The Poison Chronicles: Where Rumors of Royal Poisoning Meet Scientific Analysis
6. Henry VII of Luxembourg, Holy Roman Emperor, 1275–1313 83
7. Cangrande della Scala, Italian Warlord, 1291–1329 91
8. Agnes Sorel, Mistress of King Charles VII of France, 1422–1450 97
9. Edward VI, King of England, 1537–1553 105

10. Jeanne d'Albret, Queen of Navarre, 1528–1572   115
11. Erik XIV, King of Sweden, 1533–1577   123
12. Ivan IV, the Terrible, Czar of Russia, 1530–1584;
    His Mother, Elena Glinskaya, ca. 1510–1538; and
    His First Wife, Anastasia Romanovna, 1530–1560   129
13. Grand Duke Francesco I de Medici of Tuscany, 1541–1587,
    and Grand Duchess Bianca Cappello, 1548–1587   137
14. Gabrielle d'Estrées, Mistress of King Henri IV of France,
    1573–1599   147
15. Tycho Brahe, Astronomer and Imperial Mathematician,
    1546–1601   155
16. Michelangelo Merisi da Caravaggio,
    Artist to Italy's Elite, 1572–1610   165
17. Henry Stuart, Prince of Wales, 1594–1612   173
18. Sir Thomas Overbury, Royal Adviser at the Court of
    James I, 1581–1613   183
19. Princess Henrietta Stuart of England, Duchesse d'Orléans,
    1644–1670   193
20. Mademoiselle de Fontanges, Mistress of Louis XIV
    of France, 1661–1681, and the Affair of the Poisons   203
21. Wolfgang Amadeus Mozart, Imperial Court Musician,
    1756–1791   213
22. Napoleon Bonaparte, Emperor of France, 1769–1821   221

Part III Poison in the Modern Era
23. Scientific Advances in the Victorian Age   233
24. The Democratization of Poison   239
25. Modern Medicis: The Rebirth of Political Poison   243

The Royal Art of Living and Dying   259
Pick Your Poison   261
The Poison Hall of Fame   267
Bibliography   269
Index   279

ACKNOWLEDGMENTS

For twenty years beginning in 1995, I eagerly read news reports of the University of Maryland's annual Historical Clinicopathological Conference, where experts investigated the medical mysteries of famous dead people. Doctors became sleuths, trying to determine why, in 4 bc, King Herod the Great had gangrenous private parts; whether infected pork chops killed Mozart in 1791; and if Abraham Lincoln could have survived his 1865 assassination if he had been whisked away in a time-traveling ambulance to a modern hospital.

The conference was the brainchild of Dr. Philip A. Mackowiak, an infectious disease specialist. Currently the Carolyn Frenkil and Selvin Passen History of Medicine Scholar-in-Residence at the University of Maryland School of Medicine, he has written two fascinating books, *Post Mortem: Solving History's Great Medical Mysteries*, and *Diagnosing Giants: Solving the Medical Mysteries of Thirteen Patients Who Changed the World*. Dr. Mackowiak is the Sherlock Holmes of historical who-done-its, or—in the case of natural causes—what-done-its.

As I started to write this book, I realized I needed a physician expert at diagnosing the final illnesses of long-dead people to check my work, and who better than Dr. Mackowiak? Doctors' email addresses are easy to find, but whether they answer you in a positive manner—or at all—is another matter. Luckily for me, Dr. Mackowiak responded with enthusiasm and has been of invaluable help throughout this project. Not only did he check the entire manuscript for medical malpractice on my part, he even corrected my grammar.

I am grateful to Donatella Lippi, professor of the History of Medicine at the University of Florence, who readily answered my questions about her conclusion of arsenic poisoning in the deaths of Grand Duke Francesco I de Medici and his wife, Bianca Cappello, and provided me with scholarly articles and photographs.

A big thank-you to Professor Jens Vellev of Aarhus University in Denmark, who exhumed and studied the remains of famed astronomer Tycho Brahe. He sent me an in-depth article of his findings and cleared up my many questions about the conflicting conclusions on Brahe's cause of death.

It was a delight to work with the staff of the University of Virginia's Claude Moore Health Sciences Library, who helped me locate obscure medical journal articles on exhumations of royal personages, their modern autopsies, and the shocking results.

Many thanks to my friend Larissa Tracy, professor of medieval literature at Longwood University, for providing me with an early look at her edited collection *Medieval and Early Modern Murder*. I found particularly helpful the chapter "Poisoning as a Means of State Assassination in Early Modern Venice," by Matthew Lubin of Duke University and the University of North Carolina at Chapel Hill.

And, as always, a thousand thanks to my long-suffering husband, Michael Dyment, who over the course of my writing this book has had to listen to details of appalling illnesses, cracking open moldy coffins, and medical tests on rotten bones and ghastly mummies, often over dinner. You didn't know you were getting into this when you married me, did you?

INTRODUCTION

In 1670, at the glittering court of Louis XIV, the beautiful twenty-six-year-old princess Henrietta, duchesse d'Orléans, sips from a cup of chicory water, clutches her side, and cries out, "I am poisoned!" Her ladies undress her and put her to bed, where she vomits and soils herself repeatedly. The ceaseless pain is like a thousand red-hot knives slashing and burning her insides. She writhes in a tangle of sweat-soaked sheets, screaming. She begs God to make the pain stop. She whimpers and groans, and falls silent.

By the time the princess dies, nine horrifying hours after the initial attack, it is a mercy. Given her symptoms, it appears that she was indeed poisoned. The suspected murderer? Her husband, Philippe, duc d'Orléans, the king's vindictive brother, furious at her for exiling his male lover.

In researching my books on royal love affairs, I was intrigued by numerous such stories of the young, the beautiful, the talented and powerful, cut down before their time. For centuries, almost every death of a relatively young royal was rumored to have been caused by poison. But was it poison? Or had they all died of natural causes?

I decided to return to this absorbing topic, which so adeptly combines my love of forensic crime shows with my passion for the past. I soon found myself up to my elbows in the grisly, the astonishing, the tragic, and the hilarious. I learned how to perform a sixteenth-century autopsy and embalming—not something for the faint of heart. Wide-eyed, I read Renaissance beauty recipe books whose ingredients included mercury, arsenic, lead, feces, urine, and human fat. I dove into modern scientific papers on the exhumations of royal bodies found to be riddled with a variety of toxic materials. And I discovered the elaborate—and to us comical—poison-prevention protocols at royal courts.

As I delved into this world, I learned that palaces were bursting with many kinds of poison, not all of them deadly doses of arsenic intended to kill. Gazing at the gorgeous portraits of centuries past, we don't see what lies beneath the royal robes flashing with diamonds: the stench of unwashed bodies; the lice feasting on scalps, armpits, and private parts; the lethal bacteria from contaminated water and poorly prepared food; and the excruciating cancers eating away at vital organs. We can't smell the nauseating odors of overflowing chamber pots or the urine-soaked staircases where courtiers routinely relieved themselves. We don't glimpse the barbaric medical treatments more dangerous than the original illness itself, or elixirs designed to beautify that sometimes killed.

To bring you into this world of sublime beauty and wretched filth, I first investigate the palace poison culture of prevention, protocols, and antidotes, followed by chapters on deadly cosmetics, fatal physicians, and the royals' perilously unhealthy living conditions. I then examine twenty cases of royal personages rumored to have been poisoned, from the renowned, such as Napoleon and Mozart, to the obscure, such as a fourteenth-century Italian warlord and a sixteenth-century queen of Navarre, household names in their own time but mostly forgotten in ours.

While palace physicians were often completely baffled when it came to determining the cause of an illness and death, modern science can shed light on what really happened to our tragic princess and many others who died mysteriously. In these chapters I examine their lives, their deaths, and their exhumations and modern analyses, if these have occurred; if not, I provide a modern diagnosis of their symptoms and probable cause of death.

What I have found is that people living in terror of poison were, in fact, poisoning themselves every day of their lives, through their medicine, cosmetics, and living conditions. At Europe's dazzling royal courts, beneath a façade of bejeweled beauty, there festered illness, ignorance, filth, and—sometimes—murder.

Nor is poisoning of one's political rivals hermetically sealed in the past. As my final chapter will show, in some countries political assassination by poison is as alive and well as ever it was in the sinister royal courts of the Renaissance.

PART I

Poison, Poison, Everywhere

1

POISON from the BANQUET TABLE
to the ROYAL UNDERPANTS

Imagine a king casting his gaze over a feast of roasted meats, rich sauces, glazed honey cakes, and fine wine. Even though his stomach rumbles with hunger, he might lose his appetite when considering that anything on the table could, in fact, cause him to die horribly over the next few hours.

Were his fears unfounded? Did all those palace personages who died young and unexpectedly succumb not to poison but to natural disease undiagnosed by bewildered physicians? No, alas. While rumor incorrectly attributed many royal deaths to poison, records prove that fear of poison was more than just palace paranoia.

Italy was the beating heart of the poison trade. Both the ruling de Medici family of Tuscany and the Venetian republic set up poison factories to produce toxins as well as antidotes and test them on animals and condemned prisoners. Unlike the ancient Romans, who used plant-based poisons to murder imperial heirs and nagging mothers-in-law, Renaissance poisoners employed heavy metal poisons—the deadly quartet of arsenic, antimony, mercury, and lead.

Among the four million documents of the Medici Archives in Florence are numerous references to poison. In 1548, Duke Cosimo I initiated a plot to assassinate Piero Strozzi, a military leader who opposed

Medici rule, by slipping poison into his food or drink. In February of that year, an anonymous correspondent wrote in cipher to Cosimo, "Piero Strozzi usually stops to drink a few times during his journey." The writer requested "something that could poison his water or wine, with instructions on how to mix it."

In 1590, Cosimo's son, Grand Duke Ferdinando, suspected of having poisoned his older brother Francesco to gain the throne three years earlier, wrote his agent in Milan, "You are being sent a bit of poison, and the messenger will tell you how to use it . . . And we are pleased to promise three thousand scudi and even four to the one who administers the poison. The quantity being sent is enough to poison an entire pitcher of wine, has neither odor nor taste, and works very powerfully. You need to mix it well with wine, and if you want to poison only one glass of wine at a time, you need to take a half ounce of the material, rather more than less."

The mysterious Council of Ten, one of the main governing bodies of the Republic of Venice from 1310 to 1797, ordered assassination by "secret, careful, and dexterous means"—a clear reference to poison. In a new study, Matthew Lubin of Duke University and the University of North Carolina at Chapel Hill has identified thirty-four cases of Venetian state-sponsored political poisonings between 1431 and 1767. Eleven of the attempts failed, nine succeeded; in two cases, the intended victims appeared to have died of natural causes before consuming poison, and in twelve cases, the outcomes are not recorded. In all probability, there were many more Venetian poison attempts on political undesirables than were recorded.

The council hired botanists at the nearby University of Padua to create the poisons. Council annals include two detailed poison recipes from 1540 and 1544 that called for the following ingredients: sublimate (mercury chloride, a poisonous white crystal), arsenic, red arsenic, orpiment (yellow arsenic trisulfide crystals), sal ammoniac (a mineral composed of ammonia chloride), rock salt, verdigris (a blue or green powder from corroding copper), and distillate of cyclamen, a flower that blooms in December in Venice.

The widespread popularity of poison lasted well into the seventeenth century. Until her execution in 1659, a woman named Giulia Toffana sold poisons for fifty years in Naples and Rome, mostly to would-be widows, killing an estimated six hundred individuals. She created what became known as Aqua Toffana, a toxic brew of arsenic, lead, and belladonna that was colorless, tasteless, and easily mixed with wine, and which remained in favor long after Giulia's death. To fool the authorities, she disguised the poison as holy water in glass vials with the images of saints or put it in cosmetics containers.

In 1676, the forty-six-year-old Marie-Madeleine-Marguerite d'Aubray, marquise de Brinvilliers, was executed in Paris for using Aqua Toffana to kill her father and two brothers in order to inherit their estates. During her interrogation, she declared, "Half the people of quality are involved in this sort of thing, and I could ruin them if I were to talk." And indeed, three years later, 319 people—including many courtiers—were arrested in and around Paris, and thirty-six were sentenced to death for poisoning.

KILLING THE KING WITH CUISINE

It would only take one person to slip a little something into a king's food. Henry VIII had two hundred people employed in his kitchens at Hampton Court: cooks, scullery maids, stewards, carvers, porters, bakers, butchers, gardeners, butlers, pantlers (pantry servants), and delivery men who plucked, chopped, boiled, baked, carried, garnished, plated, scrubbed, and ran errands. Royal kitchens were food factories, pumping out hundreds of meals a day as servants trudged in and out.

With such an unsettling number of hands touching his food, what steps did a royal take to avoid ingesting poison? The earliest advice comes from the great Jewish physician, philosopher, and scholar Maimonides, who in 1198 wrote a treatise on the subject for his employer, Sultan Saladin of Egypt and Syria. He advised against eating foods with uneven textures, such as soups and stews, or strong flavors that could conceal the flavor or texture of poison. "Care should also be exercised with regards to foods . . . obviously sour, pungent, or highly-flavored," wrote Maimonides, "also ill-smelling dishes or those prepared with onion or garlic. All these foods are best taken from a reliable person, above all suspicion, because the way to harm by poison is only to those foods which assimilate the poisonous taste and smell, as well as the poison's appearance and consistency."

According to Maimonides, poison in wine was particularly dangerous and difficult to detect. "The trick is easily done by mixing the poison with wine," he wrote, "because the latter as a rule covers up the poison's appearance, taste, and smell, and speeds it up on its way to the heart. Whoever drinks wine about which he has reason to suspect that someone has tried to outwit him is certainly out of his mind."

In the late sixteenth century, the powerful minister of Spain, Gaspar de Guzmán, Duke of Olivares, was evidently well aware of the dangers of poisoned wine. According to a report in the Medici Archives in Florence, Olivares, when dining in the city of Valencia, "having taken his first drink and tasting a very unnatural flavor in the wine, he feared poisoning and jumped away from the table in a great fury asking for remedies. Meanwhile the wine steward, having heard what was going on, reassured His Excellency that the bad taste resulted from his not having rinsed the wine flask well after washing it with vinegar and salt. When the steward then preceded to drink the same wine, he [Olivares] finally calmed down."

Girolamo Ruscelli agreed with Maimonides. He wrote the 1555 book *The Secrets of the Reverend Maister Alexis of Piemont, Containing Excellent Remedies Against Diverse Diseases, Wounds, and Other Accidents, with the Maner to Make Distillations, Parfumes, Confitures, Dyings, Colours, Fusions, and Meltings*, which swept across Europe in numerous translations and editions. In a section called "For to preserve from poisoning," he noted, "You must take heed that you eate not things of strong savor, or of a very sweete taste, because that the bitternesse and stench of poisons in this maner is wont to be covered, for the over-sweet, souer, or salte thing mixed with poison, doth hide the bitternesse of it."

Ambroise Paré, physician to four kings of France, wrote in his 1585 treatise on poisons, "It is a matter of much difficultie to avoid poisons because . . . by the admixture of sweet and well-smelling things, they cannot easily bee perceived even by the skillful. Therefore such as fear poisoning ought to take heed of meats cooked with much art, verie sweet, salty, sowr, or notabley endued with anie other taste. And when they are opprest with hunger or thirst, they must not eat or drink too greedily, but have a diligent regard to the taste of such things as they eat or drink."

For thousands of years, kings hired tasters to test each dish before it reached the royal mouth. However, poisons—even a hefty dose of arsenic—don't necessarily work instantly. Contrary to what we see in film, the victim of poison didn't swallow something, grab his throat, and hit the floor dead. The length of time required for the first symptoms (abdominal pain, vomiting, and diarrhea) to appear varied greatly depending on the individual's height, weight, genetics, general health, and how much food was already in the stomach, which would slow the poison's absorption.

One of the few recorded examples of this phenomenon occurred in 1867 when a group of twenty guests sat down to a meal at an Illinois hotel and ate biscuits mistakenly made with arsenic instead of flour. One guest fell ill shortly upon rising from the table, while the others became sick over several hours, although they all consumed the arsenic at the same time. All the victims had nausea and diarrhea, but other symptoms varied, including a burning pain in the gut, a constricted throat, cramps, and convulsions. One victim had diarrhea and difficulty urinating for several weeks. None died.

Certainly, the royal family wouldn't wait at the table an hour or two after a taster tested their meal to see if he started retching—their food would be stone cold. Evidently, kings and their physicians weren't aware of this time lag and expected poisoned tasters to start gagging and vomiting immediately. They also must have relied on the taster to test for unusual flavors or textures.

According to Maimonides, it was preferable if the taster—or a host whom the king suspected of unkindly intentions toward him—took a great heaping helping of the food rather than a polite nibble. "Someone who wants to guard himself against someone else whom he suspects," the philosopher wrote, "should not eat from his food until the suspect first eats a fair quantity from it. He should not be satisfied with eating only a mouthful, as I have seen done by the cooks of kings in their presence." To prevent the poisoning of his hard-won son and heir, the future Edward VI, Henry VIII had tasters stuff their faces with the young prince's milk, bread, meat, eggs, and butter before the boy took so much as a spoonful.

By the Middle Ages, the tasting of the king's food developed into a complicated set of protocols, rituals, and safeguards. Testing began in the royal kitchen. A 1465 report of the banquet held to celebrate the

installation of George Neville as Archbishop of York described the numerous assays, or tests, of the dishes. "In the mean tyme the Sewer
goeth to the dresser," the author explained, "and there taketh assay of
every dyshe, and doth geve it to the Stewarde and the Cooke to eat of
all Porreges, Mustarde, and other sawces . . . And of every stewed
meate, rosted, boylde, or broyled, beyng fyshe or fleshe, he cutteth a
litle thereofe . . . and so with all other meates, as Custardes, Tartes, and
Gelly, with other such lyke."

When faced with any dish bearing a crust, such as a meat pie, the tasters broke the crust, dipped bread into the food below, and tasted it. By
the time the monarch received a plate of food, the resulting haggis was
not only lukewarm but may have looked more like a dog's breakfast
than a king's dinner. Servants carried the tested dishes in pompous
procession to the royal dining chamber, where they placed them on a
credenza, which takes its name from the various "credence" tests for
poison conducted there. Each servant had to eat from the dish he himself had carried, and armed guards made sure no unauthorized person
approached the food.

Anything the king drank—whether water, wine, or ale—was also
tested, of course. The taster poured a few drops of the beverage into the
"bason of assay," or testing basin, and drank it. A servant also tested
the water the king used to wash his hands before and after eating by
pouring some from the royal basin over his own hands to see if it caused
pain, itching, or burning.

But tests were not only reserved for food and drink. Servants also
kissed the king's tablecloth and seat cushion. If their lips didn't itch or
swell, they assumed the items were poison-free.

Even the king's salt was tested. The pantler scooped out a bit of salt
from its large, ornate dish and passed it to the porter to taste. The servant bringing the king's napkin from the linen closet did so by hanging
it around his neck so that he could hide no poison in its folds. According to the 1465 report, "Then the Carver taketh the Napkyn from his
shoulder and kysseth it for his assay, and delyvereth to the Lorde. Then
taketh he the Spoone, dryeth it, and kysseth it for his assay." With all
this kissing of the king's utensils, it is far more likely his royal highness
was sickened with germs rather than arsenic.

According to the 1712 edition of *État de la France*, an annual ad-

ministrative report, in his last years Louis XIV employed 324 people
to serve the royal table at the Palace of Versailles. The king generally
preferred to dine at one o'clock in his own apartments. Though he was
the only one eating, he wasn't alone. In addition to the bevy of servants
assisting him, courtiers and ambassadors stood watching him. Sometimes the king joined the court and the rest of the royal family at a
banquet where the protocol was even more stifling, and members of
the public were allowed to walk by, gaping at the sight of a monarch
chewing.

Before Louis XIV entered the dining chamber, the Officers of the
Goblet "made the trial" of tablecloths, napkins, cups, dishes, cutlery,
and toothpicks by kissing them, rubbing them against their skin, and,
in some cases, rubbing bread against the tableware and then eating the
bread. A servant even moistened the king's fine linen napkin and rubbed
his hands with it before folding it and placing it back on the king's
table. Oddly, the king thus always used a soiled, wet napkin.

At the same time, servants in the Office of the Royal Mouth in the
kitchen tested the king's food. Then each one took a dish and lined up
in pompous parade formation with butlers carrying silver batons and
guards carrying guns to make sure no one got near the food. This contingent began its long trek to the king's dining room. Leaving the royal
kitchens, they crossed a street, entered the south wing of the palace,
ascended a flight of stairs, traversed several long corridors, crossed
the upper vestibule of the Staircase of the Princes, passed the Salon of the
Shopkeepers, the Grand Hall of the Guards, the upper vestibule of
the marble staircase, and the Hall of the King's Guards before reach-
ing the first antechamber of the king's apartments. By then, we can imagine, the food was lukewarm at best. Throughout the meal, servants
at the table of trial continued shaving off bits of the king's dinner and
eating them.

Like Louis XIV, the Tudors usually ate in their private apartments,
enjoying a more relaxed atmosphere with reduced pomp and circumstance. But unlike Louis, they built small privy kitchens below the royal
apartments in their various palaces. These private kitchens offered the
advantages of warmer food, which didn't have to be carried across a
cold courtyard, and less risk of poison, as only a handful of trusted
servants came near the meals.

In all royal palaces, servants refreshed the decanters of wine and water in the king's rooms throughout the day. If he expressed the desire to whet his whistle, the Officers of the Goblet made the trial in front of him. If the king wanted a picnic on a hunt, the same servants would test his food and beverages. Never would anything, except medicine and Holy Communion, enter the royal mouth without others testing it for poison first.

The household servants had good reason to ensure the king was not poisoned or even suspected he might have been when he was, in fact, merely suffering from an upset stomach. If the royal intestines went into an uproar, the king could have any or all of these servants tortured horribly, and under such torture even the most innocent person would probably confess to a crime. Once a confession was torn out of them, along with chunks of flesh by red-hot pincers, the admitted poisoners would be executed in some awful way: hanged, drawn and chopped into quarters, or pulled apart by four horses.

Some poisoners, aware of the difficulty of poisoning the king's food with so many tasters, came up with more creative methods. On May 26, 1604, when King Henri IV of France opened his mouth to take the communion wafer from a priest, his dog suddenly grabbed the king's coat with his teeth and pulled him back. Henri moved forward again to take the host, but again the dog yanked him back. The king believed the dog was trying to warn him of something and ordered the priest to eat the wafer. At first, he refused, but the king insisted. According to a contemporary report from Venice, "When the priest had taken it, he swelled up and his body burst in twain." Since no known poison causes a body to burst in twain, the correspondent was probably exaggerating the violent effects of diarrhea and vomiting, which can certainly make one feel as if one were bursting in twain. "Thus was the plot discovered," the writer continued, "and some of the noblemen privy to it are now in the Bastille."

POISONED OBJECTS

Monarchs weren't worried only about what they consumed. They were also terrified of touching something coated with toxins, allowing the poison to enter through their skin. As Ambroise Paré, the sixteenth-century French royal physician, wrote, "Now poisons do not onely kill being taken into the bodie, but som being put or applied outwardly."

The gentlemen who made Henry VIII's bed every morning had to kiss every part of the sheets, pillows, and blankets they had touched to prove they had not smeared poison on them. The king was also quite concerned that his enemies might try to poison his son's clothing. New garments straight from the tailor were never to be put on the prince; they must first be washed and aired before the fireplace to remove any harmful substances. Before the prince donned any items of clothing— hose, shirt, or doublet—his servants tested them; either they rubbed them, inside and outside, against their skin, or they dressed a boy Edward's size in them and waited to see if he cried out that his skin was on fire.

Henry VIII decreed that no one could even touch his son without express permission. Those few who were permitted to plant a kiss on the boy's hand were first obliged to perform a "reverent assay": in other words, they had to kiss a servant's hand, after which everyone would stare at the kissed spot to see if it reddened and blistered from some poison the kisser had smeared over an antidote on his lips. Even the cushion on Edward's chamber pot was tested before he used it, though we are not sure how. Perhaps one of his servants sat on it with his bare butt and waited to see if his cheeks flamed up bright red and burning.

In 1560, Elizabeth I's secretary of state, William Cecil, concerned about a Catholic plot to poison the new Protestant queen, took extra precautions not only with the queen's food, but also with her clothing. He decreed that she was not to accept the traditional gifts to a queen— perfumed gloves and sleeves. No unauthorized person was to be allowed near her wardrobe. The royal underwear, and "all manner of things that shall touch any part of her majesty's body bare," had to be carefully guarded, tested, and examined before the queen wore them. With regard to testing the royal underpants, we can only wonder whether Elizabeth's ladies-in-waiting kissed them, rubbed them against their hands, or even tried them on to see if their private parts burned before they removed them and handed them to her majesty. Her ladies also tested new gifts of perfume and cosmetics for poison before passing them on to the queen.

And indeed, throughout Elizabeth's long life, plots abounded to poison her one way or another. In 1587, the French ambassador to England, the baron Chateauneuf-sur-Cher, plotted to have one of Elizabeth's gowns poisoned, though it seems the poison was never administered and would probably have done no harm if it had been, considering all the undergarments a lady wore.

In 1597, Spanish Jesuits hatched a plot to kill Queen Elizabeth and her favorite, Robert Devereux, the Earl of Essex. They hired Edward Squire, who worked in the queen's stables, to smear poison on her saddle pommel. Apparently, the poison had no effect because the queen always wore leather riding gloves. Squire then signed on to sail with the earl, and on board the ship he smeared the earl's chair with poison, another complete failure. The Spaniards, believing Squire to be a double agent rather than simply inept, informed the English government of his plot. The failed assassin was hanged, drawn, and quartered.

It is doubtful that any poison transferred to skin could have killed an adult. One of the few documented cases of death by cutaneous absorption of poison occurred in 1857, when an English woman thoroughly dusted her six-week-old child's entire body with what she thought was baby powder but turned out to be arsenic. The baby was not in a position to say her skin was burning, and the poison, drawn into the bloodstream through the blisters and the private parts, overwhelmed the tiny body, killing the child. Yet if an adult handled poisoned paper, cloth, wood, or other objects, the resulting burning sensation would cause him to wash off the affected area immediately, suffering nothing more than a skin rash. Due to scientific befuddlement, however, no one knew this, and ignorance always fans the flames of fear.

Some monarchs feared the very air they breathed. In 1529, Queen Marguerite of Navarre, a tiny country wedged between France and Spain, heard that a Catholic bishop was plotting to poison her by unorthodox means for her friendship with Protestants and her efforts to reform the Church. "It is reported that the monks have invented a new mode of poisoning their enemies," she wrote, "by the smoke of incense" during church service.

In 1499, as Cesare Borgia—the son of Rodrigo Borgia, Pope Alexander VI—raped and pillaged his way across Italy, some noblemen decided to poison the pope, thereby taking away Cesare's army. A

Vatican musician and steward agreed to hand a petition to Alexander so drenched in poison that the fumes would kill him as soon as he unrolled it, but the plot was discovered before it could be put into action. Similarly, in the 1670s, a group of Parisian poisoners decided to kill King Louis XIV by handing him a poisoned petition, though they were never able to get near him.

The would-be assassins left us no clues about the kind of poison they used, and they must have had difficulty creating poisoned petitions without poisoning themselves from the fumes. It is highly unlikely that any poison of the era could retain its strength on paper, or that the victim, with his nose several inches away, could inhale enough to kill him. And yet, if poison vapor were delivered effectively, it could indeed kill. Ambroise Paré correctly believed that inhaled poison was the most dangerous of all, writing, "For that poison which is carried into the bodie by smell is the most rapid and effectuall." Renaissance-era poisons that entered the digestive tract were mostly evacuated through vomiting and diarrhea, giving the victim a chance of survival, while poison fumes—a blast of the odorless, tasteless mercury, for instance—would have gone directly to the brain. It is hard to imagine, however, the faint fumes from dried poison on paper having a deleterious effect. In the case of the murderous monks swinging poisoned incense, if their plot was successful, everyone in the room would have sickened and died, including the monks themselves.

Paré described a clever way to poison the intended victim—and only the victim—by inhalation from a pomander, a perforated metal ball containing herbs or other sweet-smelling substances melted into a ball of wax, which dangled by a chain from one's belt. Every time the pomander knocked against the wearer's leg or skirt, fresh waves of sweet scent would rise. If the individual walked through a particularly noisome area, he or she would hold the ball right against the nostrils. "A certain man not long ago," Paré wrote, "when hee had put to his nose and smelled a little unto a pomander which was secretly poisoned, was taken with a Vertigo and all his face swelled and unless that hee had gotten speedie help by sternutatoria [a substance that causes sneezing, such as pepper], and other means, hee had died shortly after."

Monarchs even had reason to fear murder from their own doctors. In 1517, Cardinal Alfonso Petrucci of Siena tried to poison Pope Leo X by having his physician smear a poisoned ointment on his holiness's notoriously diseased rear end. The plot was discovered in time and the cardinal executed. In 1613, Sir Thomas Overbury died in agony after his enemies at the court of James I paid a doctor to give him a sulfuric acid enema.

The threat of poison terrified those living at royal courts because there was no way to know if a monarch had been murdered or died of a natural illness. Medical knowledge of the human body was appallingly meager. Anytime someone clutched their stomach and raced off to the nearest chamber pot, those nearby must have looked at one another in suspicion and horror.

The symptoms of poisoning from arsenic, foxglove, and death cap mushrooms have much in common: abdominal pain, diarrhea, nausea, vomiting, headaches, confusion, dehydration, coma, and death. But those suffering from food poisoning—salmonella and E. coli (bacteria that live in feces, unclean water, unpasteurized milk, and meat), and the initial symptoms of trichinosis (a parasite in undercooked pork)—experience those same symptoms. Such digestive complaints must have been common in eras of unevenly cooked meat—turned on a spit, often one half was raw while the other was dried out—contaminated wells, and no refrigeration, pasteurization, or food inspectors. The proximity of livestock increases the risk of E. coli, and all courts housed horses, cows, sheep, and pigs. Cooks rarely washed their hands, and in the days before intravenous drips to dispel the fatal effects of rapid dehydration, food poisoning could be just as deadly as arsenic.

What palace doctors didn't know was that arsenic and other poisons did not cause fever, which is a symptom of food poisoning and, particularly, malaria. That's not to say that someone with a fever couldn't be tipped over the edge with arsenic, or that someone being poisoned over a period of time couldn't die from an illness with a fever. But it is an important clue. Malaria was rampant in Italy, in particular. Roman emperors had drained many of the mosquito-breeding swamps, but they returned after the empire dissolved into chaos in the late fifth century. Many Italian cardinals, princes, warlords, and even popes died of malaria but were assumed to have died of arsenic, given all their known enemies.

Prime examples of medical malarial confusion were Pope Alexander VI and his vicious warlord son, Cesare. In early August 1503, both men dined alfresco with Cardinal Adriano Corneto in his vineyard outside Rome. On August 12, all three became violently ill, perhaps bitten by the same malarial mosquito. The pope died on August 18, but Cesare and the cardinal survived. Rumor had it the pope and Cesare had tried to poison Corneto, but the flasks of wine had gotten mixed up and they drank the poisoned wine by mistake. No one seemed to understand that it doesn't take over a week for symptoms of arsenic to appear, but it does for symptoms of malaria.

Courtiers in northern Europe were well aware of the mysterious deaths at Italian courts, along with the state-sponsored poison factories in Florence and Venice. So much so, in fact, that when a royal personage died unexpectedly, courtiers fixed suspicious stares on the nearest Italian in the entourage. A new term arose in England in the sixteenth century: someone believed to have been poisoned was said to have been "Italianated." In *The Devil's Banquet*, a 1614 collection of sermons, the English clergyman Thomas Adams argued, "It is observed, that there are sinnes adherent to Nationes, proper, peculiar, genuine, as their flesh cleaveth to their bones . . . If we should gather Sinnes to their particular Centers, wee would appoint Poysoning to Italie." In Thomas Nashe's 1594 novel *The Unfortunate Traveler*, an English earl sums up contemporary English beliefs about Italians when he calls them addicted to "the art of whoring, the art of poisoning, the art of sodomitry."

Sodomitry and whoring aside, it is difficult to judge whether Italians were more willing to tip a bit of arsenic into an enemy's wine than citizens of other countries. To be sure, documents in the Tuscan and Venetian archives prove that their rulers attempted assassination by poison on numerous occasions. But it is possible other monarchs did the same and left no archival evidence. What we do know is that an Italian in a foreign court could be hauled up on poison charges in part, at least, because of his nationality.

In 1536, an Italian courtier, Count Sebastiano Montecuccoli, was found guilty of poisoning the heir to the French throne, eighteen-year-old François, Duke of Brittany, because he handled a water pitcher the prince drank from shortly before his fatal illness. Even though the autopsy revealed abnormalities in François's lungs, the king was convinced the Italian had murdered his son and had him pulled apart by four horses. Whatever killed the dauphin, it wasn't poison, which would not have caused his high fever.

POISON AUTOPSIES

By the fifteenth century, autopsies were performed on most royal personages to determine the cause of death and, hopefully, allay the ever-present rumors of poison. Palace physicians generally had a good idea of what poisoned organs looked like, but they were also looking for evidence of natural disease that might have been the cause of death. Whatever they found, they usually called the death a natural one, reluctant to antagonize power factions at court or even send their country to war with the perceived foreign poisoners.

During the autopsy, numerous royal physicians examined the exterior of the body, all internal organs, and usually the brain for injuries or signs of illness, as do medical examiners today. But a modern autopsy relies on toxicology tests to make a determination of poison. Before the development of such tests in the nineteenth century, physicians looked for foam or blood in the mouth, an extremely bad odor emanating from the corpse, blackened nails falling off the fingers, livid spots on the skin, corrosions in the esophagus and stomach, black spots on the intestines, and congealed blood around the heart or in the stomach. The physicians were generally adept at noticing unusual changes to the organs but had no idea what they meant. If physicians conducting a postmortem discovered a substance that looked like poison in the internal organs, they gave it to a dog to see if it would start howling in agony and die.

Typical medical bewilderment occurred in 1571 when Odet de Coligny—a former Catholic cardinal who had become Protestant, married his mistress, and fled to England—died in agonizing abdominal pain at an inn in Canterbury. The turncoat cleric had been returning to France to join the Huguenot army. Rumor had it that a servant, bribed by the ardently Catholic French queen mother, Catherine de Medici, had slipped a little something into his wine. The deceased's mother howled for an autopsy, which revealed "the liver and the lungs corrupted," pointing to natural illness. But they also found spots on the stomach, a perforation of the stomach walls, and lacerated tissues.

The chief physician told the man's mother that the symptoms were the result of a corrosive agent that ate into the stomach. But in the twentieth century, physicians studying the autopsy report believed Coligny had a gastric ulcer that ruptured, allowing his stomach contents to flood his abdomen and resulting in death.

Many official autopsy reports have survived in national archives, including one from Ambroise Paré. "M. de Castellan, physician in ordinary to the king," he wrote,

and Master Jean d'Amboise, surgeon in ordinary to the king, and myself, were sent to open the body of a certain personage that one suspected of having been poisoned, because, before having supped he had not complained of any pain. And soon after supper he complained of a severe pain in the stomach, crying out that he was suffocating, and the entire body became yellow and swollen, unable to breath and panting like a dog who had ran a long distance; because the diaphragm (principal instrument for the respiration), being unable to have its natural movement, redoubled its action and thus hastened the course of respiration and expiration: then he had vertigo, spasm, and failing of the heart and consequently death. . . .

Now in truth in the morning we were shown a dead body, which was completely swollen . . . D'Amboise made the first incision, while I withdrew behind, knowing that a cadaverous and stinking exhalation would come out, this which did occur, and which all those present could hardly endure; the intestine, and generally all the internal parts were greatly blown out and filled with air; and thus we found a large quantity of blood which had escaped into the entrails and the cavity of the thorax [the chest cavity], and it was concluded that the said personage might have been poisoned.

On September 8, 1682, a physician of Lyons, France, Nicolas de Blegny, was called upon to investigate a reported poisoning. "Reported by us, master surgeons sworn," he wrote. "We went to rue des Landes, in a house which bears as sign the image of Saint Margaret, in order to visit the dead body of Suzanne Pernet, a sworn matron. Having found

all the external parts in their natural position, we then proceeded to
the opening of her body, and having commenced by the abdomen and
afterwards opened the stomach, we found it completely cauterized in
its fundus, which contained a black sandy liquid in quantity about as
much as an eggful."

The black sandy liquid and the cauterized fundus—the uppermost
section of her stomach had melted—was suspicious enough. But what
happened next gave clear proof. When de Blegny placed the organs "in
a metal vessel, they stained it, as would be done by acid and corrosive
liquids." Next, he gave "a small quantity to a dog," and it "acted on him
severely as we were able to recognize by his cries and howling, all of
which made us consider that the said Pernet had been poisoned by arsenic or sublimate [the chemical compound of mercury and chlorine],
or other such corrosive poisons of the mineral gender; in which we
were all the more confirmed by the excellent condition of all the other
intestinal parts, as much in the abdomen as in the chest and head, which
we had likewise opened, and where we found no cause for death."

2

UNICORN HORNS and ROOSTER DUNG

POISON DETECTORS and ANTIDOTES

Over the centuries, royal courts developed methods for detecting poison or, if poison had been consumed, for reversing its fatal effects. Most such methods were both medically useless and extraordinarily silly, yet they were trusted by some of the most powerful and educated people in Europe.

One of the most prized possessions of any monarch was a unicorn's horn, in part because of its rarity—only a handful of travelers to exotic places in Asia and Africa had ever reported seeing a unicorn. But monarchs cherished their unicorn horns mainly for their amazing ability to detect poison in anything nearby, either in food or drink or on garments, paper, or furniture. Royals would have been devastated to learn that their unicorn horns were, in fact, the tusks of a medium-sized Arctic whale called a narwhal, an elusive creature not discovered until the eighteenth century. Until then, sailors were surprised at how many unicorns chose to die on cold northern beaches.

Before the monarch ingested the tiniest tidbit, his tasters—in addition to testing the food and kissing the napkins and silverware—waved the horn slowly over the royal table, and sometimes dipped the horn into food and drink for good measure. The unicorn horn was believed to sweat, change color, and shake if it came near poison, although, given the horrendous tortures applied to those accused of trying to poison the king, the servants wielding it were far more likely to sweat, change color, and shake.

Many believed unicorn horns could even render poison harmless. Physicians of the Doge of Venice threw unicorn horns into the palace well so the water could never be tainted. In the 1490s, the Grand Inquisitor of the Spanish Inquisition, Tomás de Torquemada, conscious that many of the heretics he sought to root out and burn would love to slip a little something into his wine, carried his unicorn horn with him on his travels, poking it into his food and drink as a precaution.

For centuries, the cost of a unicorn horn was at least eleven times its weight in gold. Charles IX of France received an offer of 100,000 crowns for his unicorn horn, which he flatly refused. Ivan the Terrible of Russia had one worth 70,000 rubles that had been found on the Arctic coast of Siberia. Queen Elizabeth reveled in her seven-foot-long, spiral unicorn horn valued at 10,000 pounds, the cost of a decent-sized castle. Her privateer Martin Frobisher had found it on a beach on July 22, 1577, while exploring what is now northern Canada. Delighted at finding a unicorn horn so unexpectedly and so far from home, he gave it to his queen to save her from assassination attempts. As an additional precaution, the queen drank from a unicorn horn cup that was supposed to explode if it came into contact with poison. (It never exploded.)

Because of their rarity, value, and usefulness against poisons, unicorn horns were popular gifts from one monarch to another. In 1540, Sigismund I of Poland gave one to Holy Roman Emperor Ferdinand I. In 1533, Pope Clement VII bought one for the outrageous sum of 17,000 ducats, then paid thousands more to have it mounted in an impressive setting of pure gold as a gift to King François I of France. The royal jeweler Benvenuto Cellini did the work, boasting in his autobiography, "My gold mounting was one unicorn's head of a size corresponding to the horn. I had made the finest thing imaginable, for I had modelled it half on a horse and half on a stag and had added a very fine mane and other kinds of adornments."

Because of its magical protective properties, unicorn horn was used to make scepters, crowns, and royal sword hilts and scabbards. In 1671, Christian V of Denmark commissioned a new throne made en-

tirely of unicorn horn, which visitors can see today in Copenhagen's
Rosenborg Castle. Sitting on his unicorn throne, the king cheerfully
consumed whatever he wanted with no fear of poison. Christian could
build himself an entire throne of the precious material because his mer-
chants and naval captains found so many horns of what we now know
to be narwhals on Scandinavian beaches.

In the 1570s, the French royal physician Ambroise Paré decided the
unicorn horn poison protocol was useless and silly. He had seen no
proof that unicorns existed and believed that the horns were some kind
of ivory. A substance so inert, he said, could offer no medical value.
Nor did he believe that one remedy could heal the effects of so many
different kinds of poison, each of which operated uniquely on the
human body. One day Paré talked to Jean Chapelain, chief physician
of King Charles IX, about retiring the unicorn horn at royal banquets.
Chapelain replied

> that hee would verie willingly take away that custom of dipping a
> piece of Unicorn's horn in the King's cup, but that hee knew that
> opinion to bee so deeply ingrassed [ingrained] in the minds of men,
> that hee feared, that it would scarce bee impugned by reason. Be-
> sides, hee said, if such a superstitious medicine do no good, so
> certainly it doth no harm, unless it bee to their estates that buy it
> with gold or else by accident, because Princes, whilst they rely
> more then is fitting upon the magnified virtues of this horn, ne-
> glect to arm themselvs against poison by other more convenient
> means so that death oftimes takes them at unawares.

A century later, Paré was proved correct. In the 1670s, England's Royal
Society investigated a unicorn horn cup and found it completely useless in disarming poison.

At the peak of their popularity, unicorn horns were so expensive that
only monarchs could afford them. Courtiers used gemstones to warn
of poison or allay its fatal effects. Waving emerald, coral, aquamarine,
and amethyst rings over food was thought to neutralize poison, as were
stones engraved with the image of scorpions. Scorpio, a water sign in
the zodiac, was believed to have cooling properties that protected against
the gut-burning ravages of poison. Like unicorn horns, gemstones were

also ground into powder and mixed with wine and food as an antidote. Some royals had gemstones set into their drinking cups. In his
1199 treatise on poisoning, Maimonides wrote, "The best simple remedy is the emerald; it is excellent for every poison one takes and for
every poisonous animal bite. Moreover, it has the specific property of
strengthening the heart, if kept in the mouth." It is tempting to imagine
the king pushing emeralds around the inside of his mouth with his
tongue as he ate, hoping not to swallow them.

Diamonds, too, were known to absolutely confound poison. The
fourteenth-century traveler and author Sir John Mandeville wrote that
"if venom or poison be brought in the presence of the diamond anon
it begins to grow moist and sweat." We can picture guests at a royal
banquet continually checking their diamond rings for sweat as each
new dish was brought and each new glass of wine poured.

"Diamond withstands poison, tho'ever so deadly," wrote the Italian
physician Camillus Leonardus in his 1502 treatise *The Mirror of Precious Stones*, before wildly declaiming its other virtues: "[It] is a defense
against the arts of sorcery, disperses vain fears, enables the quelling of
quarrels and contentions, is a help to lunatics and such as are possessed of the devil. Being bound over the left arm it gives victory over
enemies, it tames wild beasts, it helps those who are troubled with
phantasms and the nightmare and makes him that wears it bold and
daring in his transactions."

Royals also prized the anti-toxic properties of bezoars: gallstones,
mineral concretions, and hairballs from animals' digestive tracts. They
ground them up into powder which they ingested, set them in rings
which they waved over food, and dropped them into goblets to see if
they set the wine to boiling—a sure sign of poison. Monarchs who
used bezoar stones included Elizabeth I, Charles V and Philip II of
Spain, and François I of France.

Toadstones or tongue stones were highly valued. Believed to be semi-
precious stones taken from the belly of a toad, they were usually fossilized shark teeth. These, too, were set into rings and waved over food
and drink. Sometimes they were ground into powders and mixed with
wine to deactivate toxic substances. This is one Renaissance poison
antidote that might actually have worked. When the calcium carbon-

ate in fossils is mixed with arsenic, it neutralizes the poison by mopping up the arsenic molecules in a chemical process called chelation. Today doctors use chelation to neutralize mercury, arsenic, and most heavy metals.

Some proactive monarchs took steps to prevent poisoning long before the first symptoms of diarrhea and vomiting appeared. Mithridates VI, king of Pontus, the Roman Republic's greatest enemy in the early first century bc, so feared poison that he ingested toxins every day to get his body accustomed to them. He consumed concoctions that may have included minute amounts of arsenic, wolf's bane, yew berry juice, poisonous mushrooms, and deadly nightshade, combined with bits of scorpion and viper. Having built up an immunity to such toxins, if he unwittingly swallowed a fatal dose of poison, he would have likely survived.

The effectiveness of Mithridates's potion was proven by none other than the wily seventy-two-year-old king himself, who, when surrounded by his Roman enemies, swallowed a massive dose of poison in order not to fall into their hands. Alas, the poison had no effect whatsoever; he didn't even burp. In the end, the king was forced to stab himself.

Many centuries later, European royals routinely ingested poison-prevention potions known as mithridate or theriac. These concoctions, however, generally called for nonpoisonous ingredients such as rhubarb, gentian, lavender, lemongrass, bay laurel, parsley, carrots, black pepper, cloves, wine, opium, and Dead Sea bitumen, pounded to a paste held together with honey and rolled into a pill about the size of an almond. We can only wonder how such a concoction was supposed to prevent poisoning.

Other theriac recipes included ingredients such as sulfur, garlic, charcoal, Saint-John's-wort, myrrh, and cinnamon, which offered—if not antidotes to poison—at least some health benefits. Recently, scientists have discovered that sulfur and garlic can neutralize arsenic in the bloodstream. Charcoal absorbs and filters a variety of poisons. Saint-John's-wort can aid the liver in reducing the harmful effects of thousands of dangerous chemicals. Garlic, cinnamon, and Saint-John's-wort are antibacterial. Myrrh is an antiseptic and analgesic, and one species has been proven to kill certain cancer cells. Myrrh gum alleviates the symptoms of asthma, digestive complaints, ulcers, colds, cough, and arthritis.

At least one Renaissance theriac recipe called for vipers and was proven to work against snake venom. In 1564, Ambroise Paré visited an apothecary in the French town of Montpellier to watch him cook up some theriac. The apothecary had a container full of live vipers for his recipe, and as Paré approached, one of them bit him beneath the nail of his pointer finger. Paré tied a cloth tightly around the finger, then dipped some cotton in a bottle of theriac and applied it to the wound. He had no ill effects.

In addition to its supposed virtues as an antidote, theriac was considered useful in maintaining general good health, a kind of Renaissance multivitamin. According to one fifteenth-century tract, theriac reduced swelling, healed rashes and sores, improved digestion, provided a good night's sleep, restored lost speech, strengthened weak limbs, and cured fevers, dropsy, epilepsy, palsy, and heart trouble.

Maister Alexis of Piedmont provided two recipes for simple nontoxic theriacs to be taken before every meal. Anyone in fear of poison, he wrote, would be well advised to eat "a walnut or two, two drie figs, and some leaves of garden Rue, with salt." This would prevent not only poison, he boasted, but also plague and the bite of a mad dog. Maister Alexis's second recipe called for honey, juniper berries, and a clay from the Greek isles of Lemnos or Samos called *terra sigillata*. "For in eating poisoned meat after it," he stated, "as soon as it is in your stomach there will come upon you a vomiting, so that you shall be constrained to cast up the meate and the poison together; but if there be none in your meat, the said preparative will not hurt you."

Here, at least, the Piedmontese author was on to something. Clays such as *terra sigillata* contain silicate particles, which attract the metals of metal-based poisons such as arsenic, mercury, and lead. The clay then carries them out of the body, preventing them from absorbing fully into the bloodstream.

THE MERITS OF VOMITING

Every time the king of France sat down to eat, three royal physicians stood behind him, ready to spring into action if His Highness exhibited signs of poison. Let us examine what those signs were.

According to Ambroise Paré,

> We recognize that a man has been poisoned, no matter in what way, when he complains of a great weight throughout the body, which makes him displeasing to himself; when the stomach gives him some horrible taste in his mouth, entirely different than that derived from ordinary meat, no matter how bad it may be; when the color of the face changes, being either livid or yellow, or another strange tint, and deformed; when he complains of nausea and the desire to vomit; when he is possessed of an uneasiness of the entire body, and it seems that everything about him is turned upside down.

In addition, the victim of poison suffers

> unquenchable thirst, and unexplicable torments; the tongue is swoln, the heart faints, the urine is supprest, the chest can scarce perform the office of breathing, the bellie is griped, and so great pains happen to other extreme parts that unless they bee helped, the patient will die, for presently will grow upon them, unless it bee speedily hindered, the devouring and fierie furie of the poison, rending or eating the guts and stomach, as if they were seared with an hot iron, and blood floweth out of the ears, nose, mouth, urinary passage and fundament, and then their case is desperate.

Long before blood flowed out of the ears, nose, mouth, and other parts, however, the physicians would have sprung into action. "Having knowledge that any man is poisoned," Maister Alexis stated, "the chiefe remedie is to make him vomite the poison, in giving him oile olive luke warme to drinke alone, or mixte with warm water, and if you have no oile, give him butter with hot water, or with the seede of nettles, and all these thinges purge the venim as well downward as upward, and having made him vomit divers times, you must purge him with sharpe glisters [enemas] downward, then give him water mixte with honie, and also olde wine enough to drink." He provided another recipe containing juniper berries, cloves, nutmegs, pine kernels, bits of human mummy, camphor, gentian, figs, dates, cinnamon, sweet almonds, fennel, *terra sigillata*, and emerald fragments. Yet another called for dead flies, dried and powdered, mixed with wine.

In 1562, Ambroise Paré dined in the company of some "who hated me to death for the Religion." (It is possible he was a closet Huguenot.) After eating some cabbage, he became violently ill and realized from the symptoms that he had ingested either mercury or arsenic. He made himself throw up, drank a large quantity of oil and milk to coat the lining of his digestive organs, and ate some raw eggs, which revived him. Maimonides likewise recommended immediate vomiting after consuming suspect food and praised rooster dung as one of the most effective means to bring this about. "It is said that excrements of roosters have a specific property to eliminate every poison by vomiting," he proclaimed.

Paré advised physicians to examine the vomit of a suspected poison victim, as the vomit "shows either by the taste, smell or color the kind of the taken poison. So that then by using the proper Antidote, it may bee the more easily and speedily resisted." He recommended an enema made of sheep suet, butter, or cow's milk to evacuate any poisons that have descended into the intestines.

The French royal physician described the most shocking treatment of all. "But if he bee wealthie whom wee suspect poisoned, it will bee safer to put him into the bellie of an ox, hors or mule, and then presently into another as soon as the former is cold, that so the poison may bee drawn forth by the gentle and vaporous heat of the new killed beast." Much against our will, we imagine the patient, half unconscious but wishing he were fully so, being dragged out of the stinking, oozing carcass of one animal and thrust into the steaming, bloody belly of another. But then again, if he survived that, he could probably survive anything. After vomiting, the king would be given an antidote, either ground-up unicorn horn or gemstones, or an anti-poison oil, a chemical compound developed in a laboratory.

In the late sixteenth century, King Philip II of Spain had a large laboratory at his Escorial Palace outside Madrid, though few records of it remain. Perhaps it comes as no surprise that the Medicis of Florence, widely rumored to be the craftiest poisoners on the planet, were leaders in developing poisons and their antidotes. In the 1540s, Duke Cosimo I established the *fonderie*, or laboratories, in Florence's Palazzo Vecchio

ELEANOR HERMAN   27

to create alchemical medicines such as potable gold, elixirs, distilled oils, perfumes, and medicines, and to conduct experiments in chemistry, pharmacology, and metallurgy. In July 1576, the ambassador of Ferrara, Ercole Cortile, wrote that Grand Duke Francesco spent "much of his day in making remedies against the plague, especially oils."

Rulers across Europe eagerly requested the famous Medici potions, and the grand dukes dispensed them as diplomatic gifts in caskets of walnut or ebony, divided into eight, ten, eighteen, or twenty-four compartments. These caskets contained not only the oils themselves, but also instructions on their use. Diplomatic archives abound with reports of such gifts. For instance, on December 9, 1561, Duke Cosimo sent a poison antidote to Cesare I Gonzaga, count of Guastalla. In May 1601, Grand Duke Ferdinando sent a casket of anti-poison oil to James VI of Scotland. And on April 7, 1619, the secretary at the Tuscan embassy in Spain urgently asked Grand Duke Cosimo II to send fresh theriac as well as antidotes to protect King Philip III from the poison that had been circulating at court.

As far as we can tell, the key ingredient in Medici anti-poison oil was scorpions. As Ercole Cortile reported in 1576, Grand Duke Francesco "led me into a small room with many basins full of live scorpions. He told me there were around seventy thousand, which he fed on a certain herb." Singularly unafraid of the poisonous creatures, the grand duke picked them up and plunged them into a flask containing one-hundred-year-old oil, which, he said, would be left in direct sunlight for fifty days. In July 1580, the grand duke's chemist, Niccolo Sisti, received twenty-one thousand scorpions in five consignments to manufacture poison antidotes. In 1590, the new grand duke, Ferdinando, paid a certain Gabriello d'Antonio for twenty-five pounds of scorpions to make his anti-poison oil.

In his 1593 book entitled *Hodgepodge of Various Secrets*, the Florentine apothecary Stefano Rosselli provides one of the grand duke's antidote recipes, which called for scorpions drowned in glass containers of olive oil to bake in the sun for forty days. They were then to be boiled for ten hours, the oil extracted and mixed with myrrh, rhubarb, saffron, and other plants. After another two weeks in the sun, the ointment would work "against all kind of poisons ingested by mouth, stings, and bites." He advised the poison victim to anoint the arteries of the head, around the heart and the pulse points of the arms and feet every six hours for both sexes, or more frequently according to need and the particular effects of the poison. Rosselli reported that a prisoner was given poison, then took an antidote made from this recipe and lived to tell about it. The only way to test an antidote was to poison a person or animal, watch them get sick, give them the antidote, and see if they survived.

GALLOWS GUINEA PIGS

In 1450, members of the Venetian Council of Ten wanted to try out a new poison they hoped would kill Francesco Sforza, Duke of Milan. "The substance has been prepared, to be precise," the report read, "as a small and round ball, the which, when thrown upon a fire, gives off a very subtle and pleasant smell. Whoever sniffs it, dies, and before this substance is administered out in the world . . . let a robber be found in our prisons . . . so that the experiment itself may be carried out on this imprisoned man, who is scheduled to die for theft."

Other ruling families, like the Venetians, tested poison and antidote recipes on prisoners condemned to death. In such cases, these gallows guinea pigs "volunteered"; that is, they snatched at the slight chance of surviving if the antidote worked. On December 19, 1547, Duke Cosimo sent two poison antidotes to his ambassador in Milan to give to Ferrante Gonzaga, a member of the ruling family. "The ampule of antipoison oil should be sent with instructions on how it is to be used," he wrote, "and send him a little in another ampule of that which has been tested, and which we reserve for our personal needs. Of the other, His Excellency should test it on someone condemned to death."

Even popes were not averse to such cruel experiments. The Sienese physician Pietro Andrea Mattioli wrote that in 1524, his master, the surgeon Gregorio Caravita, tested a new poison antidote on two condemned Corsican assassins, Gianfrancesco and Ambrogio, before the Medici pope, Clement VII. Both prisoners were given wolf's bane, but only Gianfrancesco was given the antidote. Both suffered three days of unbearable torment; Gianfrancesco recovered fully, while Ambrogio died.

In 1581 in Baden, Germany, a criminal condemned to hang made an unusual offer to the judge—he would volunteer to test a deadly poison on two conditions. First, that he be given a clay to eat along with the poison, and second, that he would go free if he survived. The judge agreed. The criminal consumed three-sixteenths of an ounce of corrosive sublimate, more than double the fatal dose. Five minutes later, he swallowed the same amount of *terra sigillata* stirred into wine. Physicians who observed the man for several hours reported that "the poison did extremely torment and vex him, yet in the end the medicine overcame it, whereby the poor wretch was delivered and being restored to his health, was committed to his parents."

The physicians were delighted with the result. They had just proven what had been suspected for centuries: that certain clays could act as poison antidotes, though they had no idea why.

Bezoar, on the other hand, despite its distinguished reputation, was utterly useless. In the 1570s, Charles IX of France told his physician Ambroise Paré that his bezoar stone could quell the ravages of all toxins. Paré, whom we have already seen scoff at the use of unicorn horns, also questioned the efficacy of bezoars and suggested they test the bezoar on a poor rogue sentenced to die anyway.

According to Paré, the king's provost "told him that he had in his prison a cook, who had stolen two silver plates from his master, and that the next day was to be hung and strangled. The King told him he wished to experiment with a stone which they said was good against all poisons, and that he should ask the said cook after his condemnation if he would take a certain poison; to which the said cook very willingly agreed, saying that he liked much better to die of said poison in the prison, than to be strangled in view of the people."

Paré continued:

And then an apothecary gave him a certain poison in a drink and at once the bezoar stone. Having these two good drugs in his stomach he took to vomiting and purging, saying that he was burning inside, and calling for water to drink, which was not denied him. An hour later, having been told that the cook had taken this good drug, I prayed Monsieur de la Trousse to let me see him, which he accorded, accompanied by three of his archers, and found the poor cook on all fours, going like an animal, his tongue hanging from his mouth, his eyes and face flaming, retching and in a cold

sweat, bleeding from his ears, nose and mouth. I made him drink
about one half sextier [about nine ounces] of oil, thinking to aid
him and save his life, but it was no use because it was too late,
and he died miserably, crying it would have been better to have
died on the gibbet. He lived about seven hours.

Paré performed an autopsy, which showed that the cook had died of
gastroenteritis from corrosive sublimate poisoning. As for the bezoar
stone, Paré reported, "The King commanded to burn it."

3

DYING to BE BEAUTIFUL

DANGEROUS COSMETICS

In 1603, Queen Elizabeth of England died at the age of sixty-nine, fairly ancient for the time. Her longevity must at least in part have been due to two habits considered quite strange by her contemporaries: she exercised frequently—dancing, riding at breakneck speed, and walking so fast her younger ladies-in-waiting could barely keep up with her—and ate "sparingly," according to contemporaries, which kept her slender until her death.

Fearful of swelling into a grotesque figure like her father, the morbidly obese Henry VIII, at court meals Elizabeth often jumped up after a few bites, forcing the rest of the diners to follow suit as etiquette forbade them from continuing with their meals once the queen had finished eating hers. We can imagine hungry courtiers stuffing chicken legs into their velvet pockets and raiding the kitchen after a meal with the queen. Luckily for them, she usually avoided banquets and picked at her food privately in her chambers.

As the Virgin Queen, Elizabeth didn't run the risk of dying in childbirth or suffering pregnancy complications. In fact, her only significant illness was a severe, almost fatal case of smallpox in 1562 at the age of twenty-nine, which left her skin pitted. Her efforts to hide the damage may have shaved a few years off her life. Back then, a flawless complexion was not simply a question of beauty. Blemishes of any kind were seen as proof of God's displeasure at sin, or worse, inner derangement, such as lewd sexual fantasies bubbling up from the private parts to the face. Some women filled in smallpox pits with a mixture of turpentine, beeswax, and human fat. Where to find human fat? You could buy it at your local apothecary or, cutting out the middleman, directly from the town executioner, who sliced it from the still-warm corpses of condemned criminals.

We do not know if Elizabeth ever used human fat on her smallpox scars. But after her recovery, the queen did start using on her face, neck, and chest a ceruse foundation, a pasty makeup consisting of tincture of white lead ore, vinegar, and sometimes arsenic, hydroxide, and carbonate. Applied over egg whites, ceruse filled in the smallpox pits and gave the skin a startling, almost silvery whiteness that refracted light. The English queen didn't invent the fashion but borrowed it from Italy, where it had started decades earlier. In his famous 1528 work *The Book of the Courtier*, the gallant Mantuan nobleman Count Baldassare Castiglione wrote of women who seem "to be wearing a mask and who dare not laugh for fear of causing it to crack."

Unfortunately, the lead absorbed through the skin and, over time, resulted in hair loss, muscle paralysis, mood disorders, and declining mental acuity. Ironically, it also corroded the skin, leaving blotches and pits, so that the user had to dollop on more to cover the additional damage, creating a never-ending cycle of skin damage and poison. Ceruse also dried out the skin, causing wrinkles. One contemporary remarked, "Those women who use it about their faces do quickly become withered and grey headed, because this doth so mightily dry up the natural moisture of their flesh."

In some cases, the makeup could be deadly. It killed one of eighteenth-century England's most famous beauties, Maria, Countess of Coventry. Her husband, the earl, hated the thick layers of paint she applied, and in 1752, only a year after their wedding, at a fashionable dinner party in Paris, he chased her around the dinner table with a napkin, hoping to catch her and wipe it off. Tragically for her, he capitulated, and the lovely countess was never seen again without ghastly white skin and bright red cheeks, even though she suffered horrendous headaches, swollen eyes, receding gums, loose teeth, hair loss, and tremors. In 1760, she died at the age of twenty-eight. "A victim of cosmetics," lamented the English press.

Mercury-based foundation was equally as fashionable—and poisonous. It concealed wrinkles, blemishes, and freckles and produced a radiant, translucent complexion, hiding all evidence of inner derangement, frustrated sexual fantasies, and God's wrath. Mercury absorbs easily through the skin and can cause birth defects, kidney and liver problems, fatigue, irritability, tremors, depression, paranoia, mood swings, excess salivation, black teeth, a metallic taste in the mouth, and, over time, death.

Many ladies used arsenic face powder over their mercury face paint, which gave the skin an enviable pallor. Chronic arsenic poisoning resulted in scaly skin on the palms and soles, tingling in the hands and feet, headaches, muscle weakness, confusion, respiratory inflammation, and anemia, and increased risk of cancer of the skin, colon, bladder, lungs, kidneys, and liver.

To add a bit of color over her white mask of lead and arsenic, Queen Elizabeth applied vermilion—powdered cinnabar, which contains mercury—to her cheeks and lips. In other words, every day the queen thickly coated her face with a variety of toxic materials. Unfortunately, just about all women at the English court—and many women at European courts—followed the queen's trendsetting fashions. Possibly, many Elizabethan ladies who died languishing deaths may have been killed by their cosmetics.

In addition to heavy metal poisoning, it seems the thick makeup could also cause rickets, a severe vitamin D deficiency due to lack of sunlight. In 2013, Italian researchers reported finding two sixteenth-century newborns with severe rickets in the Medici family crypt in Florence. Apparently, their mothers had absorbed almost no sunlight during pregnancy. Dressed in layers of heavy material, they coated what little exposed skin remained with thick lead-based makeup that completely blocked the sun's rays.

During the last years of her life, Elizabeth lost her appetite and deteriorated mentally and physically. She routinely erupted into temper tantrums with her ladies-in-waiting and sometimes threw cosmetics and brushes at them. The queen's godson, Sir John Harington, noticed that she "doth not now bear with such composed spirit as she was wont;

but . . . seemeth more forward than commonly she used to bear herself towards her women." While she had always taken sensible measures to ensure her personal safety, as all monarchs did, by the 1590s she had developed a strong streak of paranoia. The Jesuits, she said, were trying to assassinate her. Sir John Harington noted, "She walks much in her privy chamber, and stamps with her feet at ill news, and thrusts her rusty sword at times into the arras [tapestry] in great rage."

She became increasingly lonely and depressed as her old friends passed away. The heaviest blow came in 1601 when she had her young admirer, Robert Devereux, second Earl of Essex, executed for treason. Giovanni Scaramelli, the Venetian ambassador, reported, "She has so suddenly withdrawn into herself, she who was wont to live so gaily, especially in these last years of her life. Her days seemed numerous indeed but not now she allows grief to overcome her strength."

In her remaining two years, the queen often sat in the dark, weeping. Elizabeth Tudor, the cunning, energetic politician, had become indecisive and querulous, and seemed to be losing her grip on her power. Some contemporaries thought this was merely the result of age. Being in one's sixties back then was like being in one's eighties now, at the end of a long life with naturally diminishing physical and mental abilities. But, more recently, some experts believe that these changes in the queen's personality could have been the result of decades of cosmetic and medicinal poisoning.

Unfortunately, no autopsy was performed on Elizabeth, who was quite squeamish when it came to her body. Not only did she make her palace physicians take a solemn oath that they wouldn't perform a postmortem on her, she also strictly forbade them from embalming her. She wanted her body to be washed, dressed, anointed with sweet-smelling spices, and gently laid in a coffin filled with aromatic herbs.

She had good reason for her horror of embalming. Before the use of IVs to remove blood and inject preservative fluid, embalming was a horrifying butchery that would land anyone who tried it today in jail for mutilating a corpse. In the embalming chapter in his medical book, Ambroise Paré wrote,

The body which is to be embalmed with spices for very long continuance must first of all be [dis]embowelled, keeping the heart apart, that it may be embalmed and kept as the kinfolks shall think fit. Also the brain, the skull being divided with a saw, shall be taken out. Then you shall make deep incisions along the arms, thighs, legs, back, loins, and buttocks, especially where the greater veins and arteries run, first that by this means the blood may be pressed forth, which otherwise would putrefy and give occasion and beginning to putrefaction to the rest of the body; and then that there may be space to put in the aromatic powder; and then the whole body shall be washed over with a spunge dipped in aqua vita and strong vinegar ... Then these incisions, and all the passages and open places of the body shall be stuffed with spices ...

The herbs and spices placed in the abdominal cavity included chamomile, balsam, lavender, rosemary, thyme, cinnamon, sage, and other spices; it must have been rather like stuffing a chicken. Paré continued,

Let the incisions be sowed up and the open spaces that nothing fall out; then forthwith let the whole body be anointed with turpentine. Lastly, let it be put in a coffin of lead, sure soldered and filled up with dry sweet herbes.

Elizabeth's wishes regarding embalming were overruled, however, given that she would not be buried in a timely manner. Six of her ladies-in-waiting had to sit next to the coffin in shifts, twenty-four hours a day, for over a month until her successor, James I, could travel to London from Scotland and make funeral arrangements. Perhaps in deference to the late queen's wishes, the embalmers did a perfunctory job. One night, an explosion ripped open the casket with a deafening crack, spewing foul-smelling gases and sending the women screaming from the room. To put a positive spin on the situation, they agreed "that if she had not been opened, the breath of her body would have been much worse."

Queen Elizabeth and other ladies of the time sought not only white faces, but white hands as well. Fortunately, custom did not decree that they slather on more poison. It did, however, require them to soak their hands in fresh blood. During the royal sport of hunting, when a kill was made, the ladies raced up to the dying creature, ripped off their gloves, thrust their hands into the pulsating wounds and organs, and rubbed the blood into their skin. Blood was used to remove warts, as in one of Maister Alexis's recipes. "When you kill a hogge," he wrote, "let him that hath the warts receive the blood even hot upon the place whereas the wartes be, and as soone as it drie let him washe it off, and if it be a woman that hath these wartes, she muste take the blood of a sowe, and she shall be healed and rid of them." The fifteenth-century medical author Jerome of Brunswick advised those wishing for thicker hair to take the blood of a thirty-year-old man, "of nature rejoicing, of mind fair, clear, and wholesome from all sickness," and either rub it on the scalp or drink it, preferably in the middle of May.

Ladies who desired darker eyebrows and eyelashes used an oil-based mixture of kohl, which was made of either lead or antimony (a cousin of arsenic) smelted from its ore, or of antimony sulfide, also known as stibnite. Or they combed their lashes and brows with a lead comb dipped in vinegar, which reacted with the lead and allowed it to leach out.

To make their eyes sparkle and look bigger, women used drops of belladonna, a plant also known as deadly nightshade, a favorite poison among the ancient Romans. Over time, this practice resulted in visual distortion, increased heart rates, and poisoning. For white teeth, Maister Alexis provided a recipe for "a noble and excellent powder" that contained grain, pumice stone, aloe, vinegar, honey, cinnamon, pearls, scrapings of ivory, quinces, and walnuts crushed into a paste and cooked with silver or gold foil. "Rub your teeth with your finger or some linen cloth, taking of the saide powder upon it . . . A beter thing cannot be found," he boasted, good enough "to present to a queene or princesse." Not only was silver and gold foil poisonous, but the abrasive powder, in taking away the stains, also removed tooth enamel.

Urine was believed to have a cleansing effect. According to the 1675 work *The Accomplisht Ladys Delight in Preserving, Physick, Beautifying, and Cookery*, urine was "very good to wash the face withal, to make it fair." In the sixteenth century, the English surgeon William Bullein claimed that those "whose faces be unclean"—which probably refers to acne—should wash their skin with distilled water of honey "mixed with strong vinegar, milk, and the urine of a boy." Maister Alexis provides us with another interesting recipe to remove warts.

"Take earth and knead it with dogs pisse," he advised, "and laie it upon the warts and they will drie up and consume awaie."

As disgusting as these recipes sound to us today, it should be noted that urea—a component of urine—is used in many modern skin creams.

Mercury face treatments were admittedly less disgusting than urine but far more dangerous. *The Accomplisht Ladys Delight* advised those suffering from an "inflamed face" to mix mercury, bay oil, and spit taken from a fasting person, and rub it all over the face. "Proved true," it added. To fade freckles, ladies rubbed on a paste of white mercury mixed with white tartar and bitter almonds or a cream of lead sulfate.

Many women today have chemical peels (which contain potential carcinogens) for a fresher, more radiant skin. Centuries ago, noblewomen peeled their skin with a mercury-based potion that they left on for eight days. Maister Alexis has provided us with an astonishing recipe for a mercury face mask involving eggs, vinegar, and turpentine mixed together in a lead dish—which would have caused the lead to leach into the mixture—added to onion, quicksilver, and lemons. He warned the reader, "Now you may not take it too soone from your face . . . but let it work its operation, and at the ende of eight daies take it off." The removal instructions advised the woman with the mercury face mask to boil a mixture of wheat bran, mallow, violet leaves, bean pods, bread crumbs, and honey, and then lean over the pot with a blanket over her head to trap the steam on her face. Sufficiently moistened, she was to rub the mask off with bread crumbs.

Having worn a poison face mask for eight days straight, well might we wonder about the state of our skin. However, the good Maister insisted, "You shall see that skin which was roughe, thicke, and rude, shalbe changed and altered into a fine, faire, and delicate skin. But beware that in eight daies after you go not abroade in the open aire, or to nigh the fire, least the new, fine, tender and delicate Skine, should be burned, or take any hurte." He added, "This is a good Secrete."

Another of Maister Alexis's recipes for *aqua argentata*, or silvered water used as a lotion, promised to make "a white, ruddie and glistering face." It called for mercury sublimate mashed in a mortar and mixed with liquid mercury and strong white vinegar. After sitting for eight days, it was mixed with twelve or fifteen crushed pearls, ground-up gold or silver, camphor, bezoar, and talc. This mixture was left in the sun for forty days, then combined with eggs, turpentine, and lemon rind. "And so it will be an excellent thing," he boasted, "to give to a Queene."

For pimples, the good Maister highly recommended ox dung. "In the month of Maie," he wrote, "when Oxen goe to grasse, or bee at pasture, ye shall take of their dunge, not too freshe, nor too drie, then distill it faire and softlie into some vessel or glasse, of the which dunge will come a water, without savour or evil stench, which will be verie excellent good, to take off all manner of spots or blemishes in the face, if you wash with it morning and evening."

NOSEBLEED WIGS AND TOXIC TRESSES

In the Elizabethan era, most Englishwomen imitated their queen, and so red hair was the height of fashion. Court ladies used a powder made of sulfur and safflower petals to color their wigs. Unfortunately, the sulfur was highly toxic and caused headaches, nausea, and nosebleeds.

For those hoping to toss aside their nosebleed wigs, there were recipes to dye hair reddish-blond. Maister Alexis provided us with one that included poisonous and caustic ingredients "which comforteth the braine and memorie." The result, he wrote, was "faire haire and glistering like gold." However, the good Maister added ominously, "Remember to use in all things a discretion and diligence at the first when you use any receipte, as for an example on this confection, you must take heed that the lie be not too strong, least that the said ointment (which I tell you is very strong) eate and consume your hair." Indeed, we are left to ponder if the lady using this recipe of antimony, lye, red vitriol, rock alum, and saltpeter, all of which have toxic qualities, was deeply disappointed, and not just by illness and death. Quite possibly, instead of glistering hair, she had none at all.

Throughout time, women have wanted luxuriant thick tresses, though the means of obtaining them have certainly changed. The 1675 *Accomplisht Ladys Delight in Preserving, Physick, Beautifying, and Cookery* recommended "ashes of Goats-dung mingled with oyl" to anoint the head. Men combating baldness mixed rat droppings with honey and onion juice and rubbed it on their bald spots. For covering gray hair, the 1561 Italian best seller, *The Secrets of Signora Isabella Cortese*, written by a female alchemist, recommended, "Take four or five spoons of quicklime in powder, two pennyworth of lead oxide with gold and two with silver, and put everything in a mortar and grind it in ordinary water; set it to boil as long as you would cook a pennyworth of cabbage; remove it from the fire and let it cool until tepid. And then wash your hair with it." Maister Alexis recommended a toxic dye "for to make a mans beard blacke. Take aqua fortis [nitric acid] and a pennye weight of fine silver and melt it in the water by the fire and anoint the beard."

ARSENIC AND OLD LICE

In centuries past, lice were a perennial problem from the filthiest hovel to the most magnificent palace. In his book *A Treatise on the Diseases of Children*, the seventeenth-century English physician Robert Pemell recommended applying to the scalp a mixture of arsenic, quicksilver, and white hellebore (a deadly flower), or combing the hair with strong mercury water and arsenic. Ambroise Paré advised lousy people to anoint their heads with a mixture of quicksilver and butter. For body lice, fleas, and bedbugs, he recommended the patient wear a cloth strip smeared with mercury and hogs' grease directly on the skin at the waist like a belt. The mercury would have poisoned the insects, and the grease would have smothered them, though the rank odor of the strip would not have endeared its wearer to those downwind.

Arsenic was used not only to remove lice from hairy body parts, but also to remove the hair itself. We can assume that moustaches and chin hair have plagued the fair sex ever since they cooked up mastodon meat in caves. And, while in centuries past a lady's arms and legs were always covered by heavy material except in the boudoir, some women still liked smooth legs and underarms.

Maister Alexis provided us with several depilatory recipes. One of them, "An Ointment to make the Hairs fall from any Place of the Body," calls for mixing eight egg yolkes, an ounce of arsenic sulfide, egg whites, and lye. "Anoint the place from the which you will have the haires to fall," he instructed, "and leave the ointment so upon it the space of a quarter of an hour or a little more: then wash the place with warme water, and all the haire will fall off." As well as some of the skin, we must assume. He saves his most important instructions for last: "You must note that the haire will not fall awaie, but when the Moone decreaseth, that is to saie, in the quarter of the wane."

THE COMPLEXION ELIXIR THAT KILLED
A ROYAL MISTRESS

Nineteen years older than her royal lover, Diane de Poitiers, the strawberry-blond mistress of King Henri II of France, went to extreme lengths to stay youthful. She ate sparingly and rode and swam frequently. But her main concern was a smooth, white complexion. She bathed in asses' milk, a known exfoliant, and always wore a black velvet face mask when outside. The historian Pierre de Bourdeille, Sieur de Brantôme, who pegged her at a few years older than she actually was, wrote, "I saw her at seventy years of age, beautiful of face, also fresh and also pleasant as she had been at thirty years of age . . . and especially she had a very great whiteness without any make-up . . . Every morning, she used some drinks made up of drinkable gold and other drugs which I do not know given by good doctors and subtle apothecaries." When the once all-powerful royal mistress died aged sixty-six in 1566, no one thought much of it. Henri II had died seven years earlier in a jousting accident, and his vengeful queen had exiled her rival to the boonies, the château of Anet in Normandy. Plus, Diane was quite elderly for the time and had been unwell for a while.

In 2008, French researchers set out to find Diane's remains. But those hoping to examine the corpses of French royals are at a distinct disadvantage. The Basilica of Saint-Denis, just outside Paris, had been the repository of royal bodies since the seventh century, each one reverently laid to rest with great pomp in a hallowed tomb. But in August 1793, French revolutionaries—we can envision them waving pitchforks—cracked open the graves, plucked jewelry off corpses, threw the bones into outside trenches, and covered them with lime. In 1817, the French royal family, now back on the throne, ordered the remains of their ancestors exhumed, but all that survived intact from the trenches were the lower portions of three corpses. The remaining bits and pieces of 158 other unidentified bodies fit into two ossuaries in the crypt.

Between 1793 and 1795, revolutionaries raided the tombs of the rich and noble across France. On June 18, 1795, inside Diane's lead coffin they found her corpse perfectly preserved, wearing an ornate ceremonial gown. The mummified remains of her two grandchildren rested with her. The tomb raiders dragged the coffin outside the church, where they stripped off the corpses' clothing and jewelry. In the hot sun the corpses quickly turned black, to the horror of onlookers. Before throwing the bodies into a hole near the church, one man grabbed Diane's hair—the entire scalp ripped right off her head—and started clipping off locks as souvenirs of the momentous occasion. Cutting hair from individuals both living and deceased was a popular custom; the locks were kept as mementoes, usually preserved in a locket or ring. Some of Diane's hair ended up under glass at her nearby château of Anet.

When French archaeologists, paleontologists, and pathologists excavated in the area where Diane had reportedly been thrown, they first found the complete skeletons of two children aged two and six—her grandchildren, they surmised. Nearby they discovered a heap of brown bones composing about 40 percent of an adult human skeleton. The right tibia and fibula had been broken in one blow and healed quite nicely. Diane had broken a leg twice in her life while riding, once the year before she died, and in another incident twenty years earlier. This fracture was the earlier one. The later break—which was set by Ambroise Paré—had been on the missing left leg.

Scientists were unable to extract DNA from the bones. But Diane's identity was confirmed by a computer superimposition of large pieces from the front of the skull—the cheek and jaw areas—over the last portrait of Diane: an exact match. Next, they examined the lock of her hair in the château. The archaic custom of keeping hair as mementoes is a boon to modern research, especially in those cases where bodies cannot be examined, because DNA can be extracted from hair if not too decayed. Moreover, mercury, lead, arsenic, and other heavy metals accumulate in the keratin of hair, which can be scanned for evidence of chronic poisoning.

Every human body has trace amounts of gold, and sixteenth-century courtiers would have had substantially more gold than we do today due to eating with gold utensils and wearing gold-embroidered clothing. But Diane's hair contained gold 250 times more than expected, along with a dangerously high mercury content. One symptom of chronic gold poisoning is thin hair: the hair in the locket was much thinner than normal, even for an older woman. Another symptom is brittle bones, which may have resulted in her leg fractures. Such high levels of toxicity would also have damaged her kidneys, caused neurological disease, and inflamed her large and small intestines. In short, it is probably what killed her.

The researchers also tested the ground around Diane's remains. Horrifyingly, it was significantly contaminated with gold that had leached out of her body as it decayed.

Maister Alexis provides us with a recipe that may have been the one used to make Diane's deadly decoctions: "To dissolve and reduct gold into a potable licour, which conserveth the youth and health." The instructions are complex and include twenty-four-carat gold foil distilled with lemon juice, wine, and other ingredients. At one point, the concoction is put in a clay pot and set in a kiln or glazier's furnace for two or three days to cook. Later, it is heated in an alembic vessel for ten or eleven days. "In the bottome of the vial," Maister Alexis stated, "the gold will remaine dissolved into licour most precious, which you must keepe in some little glasse well stopped. Thus doing ye shall have a right natural and perfect potable golde, taken everie month once or twice . . . verie excellent to preserve youth and health."

Doctors who examined the royal mistress's bones believe, however, that she didn't drink the gold once or twice a month, as Maister Alexis recommended, but every day, as Brantôme indicated, in a desperate effort to look young. The deadly daily potion did, at least, provide her with the ghastly white skin she wanted. She had severe anemia caused by the reduced production of red blood cells.

4

MURDEROUS MEDICINE

MERCURY ENEMAS *and* RAT TURD ELIXIRS

A ny royal feeling a bit under the weather would have been well advised to bar his door from palace physicians, who prescribed poison on a regular basis. Medications contained lead, mercury, arsenic, antimony, gold, and silver. The sicker the patients became, the more heavy metal medicines they took, and the sicker they became. Many unexplained royal illnesses and puzzling symptoms must have been caused by the very medicinal treatments designed to heal them. Well might we laugh at the medical beliefs of the time if they hadn't killed so many millions. Learned Renaissance physicians followed the practices of the fifth-century bc Greek physician Hippocrates, and those later worthies who furthered his theories, such as Galen, physician to several second-century ad Roman emperors, and the eleventh-century Persian scientist Avicenna.

The body, they believed, had four humors: blood, phlegm, black bile, and yellow bile, which emitted vapors that rose to the brain and affected a person's health, personality, and morality. An imbalance in these humors caused illness. Disease could be cured through diet, potions, or draining the excessive humors through bloodletting, projectile vomiting, sheet-soaking sweats, blistering, and hearty explosions of diarrhea.

Since every individual was thought to have a predisposition to one humor more than the others, upon meeting a new patient the physician would first conduct a kind of Renaissance Myers-Briggs test. People with sanguine humor were cheerful and outgoing, their temperament and health boosted by a predominance of blood. Cowardly individuals cooked up too much phlegm. Melancholy, lazy creatures produced an overflow of black bile. And angry, red-faced souls with the choleric humor were bubbling over with yellow bile. Each humor was either hot or cold, dry or wet, and associated with one of the four elements (earth, water, fire, and air) and influenced by three of the zodiac signs.

Foods were labeled hot or cold and dry or wet. A phlegmatic person with naturally cold, wet humors could achieve humoral balance by eating food with hot, dry humors such as ginger, pepper, onions, and garlic. Those of sanguine humor should eat sparingly of meat, onions, leeks, and figs. Melancholic individuals should eat milk hot from the udder, blanched almonds, and raw egg yolks, and drop hot molten dollops of gold or silver into their wine and ale. A choleric person was advised to always have something in his stomach, otherwise "unsavory fumes and vapors do issue oute therof, consuming all naturall moysture, fumosities and stinkynge vapours ascendynge up to the heed," according to *The Castle of Health*, a 1539 English medical book by Sir Thomas Elyot.

Humors and the foods that fed them were also believed to control sex and fertility. Red meat, sugar, and wine were thought to boost sexual desire. Foods that produced gas, such as beans, were consumed in the hope that they would pump up a penis at the required moment, though the resulting flatulence might put an end to the partner's interest. Women, who were composed of cold, wet, phlegmatic humors, were sexually insatiable for the hot seed of men. But as sex just increased a woman's humors, too much would render her infertile as her uterus would become too cold, wet, and slippery to hold on to the hot seed. Women of all humoral natures who did not have regular sex were tormented by "naughty vapors" rising to the brain, resulting in pimples and insanity. If diet alone didn't balance the dangerous fumes, doctors recommended wearing a nightcap to bed with a hole in the top to allow them to escape.

Colors, too, had their humors. Red was believed to generate heat in cold people, and blue to cool the vapors of hot people. Depending on a person's natural humor and symptoms, physicians would wrap them in blankets of a particular color in the hope of achieving humoral balance and thereby vanquishing the illness.

To counter hot, dry humors, physicians prescribed potions including liquid silver or quicksilver, with their cold, fluid shimmer. To reduce the cold wetness of black bile, they called for remedies including the dry, hot, toxic mineral sulfur or liquid gold. Jewels, too, were believed helpful in balancing the humors, and many medicines included powdered pearls, emeralds, coral, diamonds, sapphires, rubies, turquoise, and amethysts.

Bloodletting was the most common form of medical treatment for people of all humors. Until William Harvey's groundbreaking book *On the Motion of the Heart and Blood* came out in 1628, physicians did not know that blood flows constantly through the body. They believed that blood could stop moving, and after twenty-four hours of circulatory immobility, evil humors would fester within it. Bleeding was seen as the way to get things going and expel the excremental humors.

Strangely, even illness itself was seen as good for the health in that it rid the body of pernicious humors. The late-Elizabethan historian Sir John Hayward wrote in *The Life and Raigne of King Edward VI* that physicians were delighted when the fourteen-year-old monarch had an attack of smallpox immediately after recuperating from measles. The "poxe," Hayward explained, "breaking kindly from him, was thought would prove a meanes to cleanse his body from such unhealthfull humors, as commonly occasion long sickness or death." Similarly, when the infant son of Philip IV of Spain had a boil dripping discharge from below his right ear for three weeks, the doctors called it "a laudable pus" that would "remedy a worse evil."

Lice infestations, too, were seen as beneficial. In 1650, the physician Robert Pemell wrote, "If lice be only in the head, in many it preserves their health, because they consume much excrementious humors."

Medicine was inextricably bound to astrology. In 1475, a Dominican monk, Thomas Moulton, advised in a treatise reprinted throughout the following century, *This is the Myrour or Glasse of Helth*, that no physician could cure an illness without a solid knowledge of the planets and stars. Many believed that certain illnesses were, in fact, the result of malign astrological influences. Plague, for instance, was caused by "vaporous fumosities and humors the which that are corrupt and drawn from the earth beneath by the attractive virtue of the bodies that be above," according to Moulton.

Medicine wasn't medicine per se, but a kind of philosophy bordering on theology. Any physician skeptical of this theory was labeled a medical heretic. The early medieval Persian scientist Avicenna wrote that his medical principles were eternal and immutable, and if experience contradicted them, the problem lay in the "imperfect" world.

Physicians operated in the rarified stratum of pure theory and usually spent more time with dusty books than patients. They certainly never performed operations, as they had taken the Hippocratic oath to do no harm, and slicing someone open with a knife was clearly harmful. They left the butchery of operations to surgeons, a much lower caste of medical practitioner, who consulted with an astrologer for the most auspicious day to perform the operation. Physicians did, however, study the patient's urine for signs of humoral imbalance—color, clarity or cloudiness, odor, and sediment. The medical community believed that urine was an expulsion of liquid from the blood and had, therefore, the same characteristics.

Each morning, four physicians clad in long, fur-sleeved gowns and black velvet caps visited Henry VIII. They carried bladder-shaped flasks that they filled with the king's urine and held up to the light for inspection.

Philippus Aureolus Theophrastus Bombastus von Hohenheim, known to history as Paracelsus, was a temperamental sixteenth-century Swiss physician who scorned most of his fellow practitioners. He wrote in disgust, "All they can do is to gaze at piss," and believed that "theory should be derived from practice." Paracelsus jeered at physicians, calling them "cushion-sitters," "piss prophets," and "high asses." "They think that their long necks and high judgement reach right unto heaven," he scoffed. Paracelsus traveled the world experimenting with new treatments and remedies. After decades of study and experimentation, he realized that "Nature is the physician, not you." He advised physicians to keep wounds clean, prescribe a healthful diet, and let nature take its course without dangerous interventions. Naturally, physicians erupted in outrage at his theories.

It is safe to say that apothecaries—the pharmacists of the day—may have killed as many patients as physicians. There were no laws concerning the medications dispensed, no tests for purity or harmful ingredients, and no expiration dates. In the 1520s, the German physician and author Cornelius Agrippa wrote that apothecaries who "minister one thing for another, or else make medicine of rotten, stale and moldy drugs, do oftentimes give a deadly drink instead of a wholesome medicine." Alarmingly, physicians and apothecaries often worked together, the one prescribing expensive concoctions, the other selling them, and both of them splitting the profits. "Physicians garbed in scarlet hats and miniver fur are in league with apothecaries," Paracelsus fumed. The seventeenth-century English physician Nicholas Culpeper called apothecaries "ignorant and avaricious retailers of medicine."

While the wealthy poisoned themselves with medical concoctions, the poorer sort relied on many harmless ingredients we have in our kitchens today, some of which were actually helpful in curing illness. Honey, for instance, is an excellent antiseptic, effective in treating wounds and burns. Willow forms the basis of modern aspirin. Mint helps calm gastric ailments, and pomegranate reduces worm infestations. Garlic boosts the immune system, reduces blood pressure and cholesterol levels, and reduces heavy metal toxicity. Lemons are loaded with vitamins and minerals and in some cases can detoxify the liver and kill intestinal parasites; they are often used today in colonic cleansing. Vinegar is an antioxidant with antimicrobial properties, and white wine can be an effective antiseptic on wounds.

No treatment was complete without a hefty dose of religious ritual: prayer, fasting, confessing sins, and helping the poor. Seeing this, God would surely look kindly on the sick person and generously offer a healing. The Spanish royal family, which held the mortal remains of saints in high regard, took such superstitions to drastic lengths. For centuries, whenever a member of the royal family was gravely ill, doctors would remove saintly body parts and entire corpses from churches and monasteries and put them in bed with the invalid. We can imagine a dainty young princess, waking from a fever and turning her head to see a grinning skull with shreds of desiccated skin and a mop of black hair lying next to her, staring at her with empty eye sockets.

But if that didn't kill her, nothing would.

For thousands of years until the late nineteenth century, physicians used heavy metal poisons to cure a variety of skin ailments. In 1585, French royal physician Ambroise Paré wrote that to cure skin ulcers, "one should apply a plate of lead rubbed and whitened with quicksilver," a remedy that included not one but two poisons. For venereal knots on bones, he cut open the muscle and smeared mercury directly on the bone. For ringworm, a fungal infection, he mixed up an ointment of lead and mercury. "Put into plasters," he wrote, "quick-silver assuageth pain, hindering the acrimonie of pustules and cholerick inflammations."

Paracelsus recommended rubbing an arsenic-based mixture on rashes and lesions. Maister Alexis treated hemorrhoids with a concoction of mercury ore, myrrh, and rose oil, though he thought sores on the nose were better healed with powdered lead and myrtle oil.

These days, it's unthinkable to apply excrement—human or animal—to an open wound or—even worse—to ingest it. But while modern doctors shudder at the thought, many Renaissance physicians advised their patients to do exactly that. Maister Alexis recommended "for him that spitteth blood by having some vaine of his breast broken," to "take mice dung beaten into powder as much as will lie upon a groate [an English coin], and put it into half a glasse ful of the juice of plantain, with a little Suger, and so give the patient drinke thereof in the morning before his breakfaste, and at night before he goe to bed." For kidney stones or bladder infections, he advised his patients to drink ox dung mixed with radishes, white wine, strawberry juice, lemon juice, sugar, and honey. Those suffering from nosebleeds should thrust hog's dung, still warm, up the nose. Human excrement, dried and powdered, was blown into the eye to cure ailments.

In the 1660s, Thomas Willis, the richest doctor in England, recommended treating lung ailments with drinks made of the dung of horses, cocks, oxen, or pigeons. The good doctor thought highly of smearing an ointment of dog turds and almond oil on the chest. He concocted beverages of sheep and goose dung for patients suffering from jaundice or handed them nine live lice to swallow. Oddly, he wrote that "merely pissing upon horse dung while it is hot has helped many jaundiced patients," though one wonders how he reached such a conclusion. He advised eating rat droppings as a surefire remedy for constipation, probably because the body would react quickly and violently to rid itself of the harmful substance.

Royal physicians lauded the virtues of dead birds. Dead pigeons, roosters, and other birds, cut in half, were often applied still bleeding to the heads and feet of patients to draw out their evil humors. English physicians used this remedy in 1612 on Henry, Prince of Wales, and in 1685 on King Charles II, both of whom died. It couldn't have been pleasant for a sick person, propped up on pillows, to watch his doctor bloodily butchering shrieking birds next to the bed. Sometimes the dead birds weren't removed in a timely manner but left to putrefy, which must have caused not only stench, but further infection. On September 22, 1689, an English physician named Dr. Cotton applied a dead pigeon to the head of one Mrs. Patty, who was suffering violent convulsions. It stayed on her pillow for five days. Rotting.

In the mid-sixteenth century, Jean Fernel, the royal physician of Catherine de Medici, queen of France, stated that "eating the still palpitating heart of a swallow confers memory and intelligence," a kind of daily vitamin against diminishing mental acuity.

No matter what century you live in, when your intestines turn to concrete, potent purges are required to get things flowing. No laxative is more potent than mercury in the form of quicksilver, which is usually not toxic when ingested. Perhaps only one-tenth of 1 percent is absorbed into the bloodstream, while the rest is voided in the stool. As Ambroise Paré wrote so descriptively in 1585, "It opens and unfolds the twined or bound up gut and thrusts forth the hard and stopping excrements." To cure constipation, he recommended giving a pound of quicksilver at a time to a puppy, collecting it when it came out the other end, boiling it in vinegar, and drinking it.

More than two centuries later, when Lewis and Clark explored the American West in 1804, the expedition's main diet was dried strips of beef. Not surprisingly, the party of thirty-three men suffered shocking constipation. With great foresight, they brought along laxative pills with a 60 percent mercury content called "thunder-clappers," which, true to their name, did the job. Because mercury doesn't dissolve in soil, modern historians have discovered many of the expedition's campsites by finding the areas they used as a latrine, giving new meaning to the term "toxic waste."

In the early eighteenth century, a new form of laxative known as the perpetual pill became popular. A pellet of antimony, a substance closely related to arsenic, was filled with a ball of mercury mixed with sugar and ingested. The resulting irritation to the gut caused rapid and gratifying blasts. The pellet was fished out of the chamber pot, washed off, refilled with mercury, and used again. Some of these pellets were passed down in families for several generations, a tradition that required an intestinal fortitude all its own.

A NIGHT WITH VENUS, A LIFETIME WITH MERCURY

In March 1493, the physician Ruy Diaz de Isla examined Christopher Columbus and his crew when they arrived in Barcelona fresh from the New World to report on their voyage to King Ferdinand and Queen Isabella of Spain. De Isla noted that several sailors suffered from a strange new malady common to the indigenous peoples of the islands they had visited. The captain of the *Pinta*, Martin Alonso Pinzón, died of the disease shortly after his return. Many of the sailors chalked up the illness to the difficulties of a long sea voyage to exotic places. Soon, however, it began to spread in Barcelona.

In August 1494, King Charles VIII of France led his army of fifty thousand soldiers into Italy with the goal of capturing Naples, which was defended mostly by Spanish mercenaries, some of whom had returned with Columbus the previous year. The French forces soundly trounced Naples in early 1495 and, while occupying the city, indulged in debauched celebrations with the very women who, we can assume, had also been friendly with the Spanish soldiers. Within a few weeks, the French army suffered from a new and terrible disease, and many soldiers became so ill they were unable to fight. Those who survived went home and spread the illness.

The Spanish and Italians called the new illness "the French disease," though the French referred to it as "the Neapolitan disease." The Russians called it "the Polish disease," and the Turks dubbed it "the Christian disease." In 1530, the Italian physician Girolamo Fracastoro invented an origin story for the illness involving a shepherd afflicted with it as punishment for insulting a god. The shepherd's name was Syphilis.

There is some controversy as to whether syphilis was brought to Europe from the New World. In the twentieth century, scientists found some fifty pre-Columbian European skeletons with syphilitic-type bone lesions. Had syphilis been lurking in Europe for centuries, possibly millennia, and then flared into a major epidemic in 1495, its timing with Columbus's return coincidental? Had his men been suffering from some other ailment? The question remains unanswered, though several diseases—leprosy, for instance—can produce a bone pattern similar to that of syphilis.

For the first few decades after its appearance in Naples, syphilis had an extraordinarily high mortality and infection rate, probably because the population had no immunity against it. The first sign was genital lesions, followed by fever, body rash, and joint and muscle pain. A few weeks or months later, large, foul-smelling, and excruciatingly painful sores appeared all over the body. Muscles and bones throbbed, especially at night, when the sufferers screamed in agony for hours. The sores became ulcers that could eat through flesh and muscle to reveal the white of bone, and could destroy the nose and lips. They often extended into the mouth and throat. Ultimately, syphilis caused blindness, insanity, and death.

The German religious reformer Ulrich von Hutten contracted syphilis around 1510 and described the experience of those who suffered from it in a treatise, *On the French Disease*. "They had Boils that stood out like Acorns," he wrote, "from whence issued such filthy stinking Matter, that whosoever came within the Scent, believed himself infected. The Color of these was of a dark Green, and the very Aspect as shocking as the Pain itself, which yet was as if the Sick had lain upon a Fire." Hutten claimed the disease was caused "through some unwholesome blasts of the Air, which happened about that time, the Lakes, Fountains, and even the Waters of the Sea were corrupted, and the Earth for a large Tract as it were poisoned thereby . . . The Astrologers, deriving the Cause from the Stars, said, That it proceeded from the Conjunction of Saturn and Mars . . . In Women," he continued, warming up to the subject, "the Disease resteth in their secret Places, wherein are little pretty Sores, full of Venomous Poison, being very dangerous for such as unknowingly meddle with them." Hutten, religious reformer though he was, paid a high price for his meddling, dying of syphilis at the age of thirty-five.

Writing later in the sixteenth century, Ambroise Paré had a better idea of the source of infection. He wrote that syphilis "may bee referred to God, as by whose command this hath assailed mankind, as a scourge or punishment to refrain the too wanton and lascivious lusts of unpure whoremongers . . . A woman taketh this disease by a man, casting in her hot, open and moist womb." Or, as one sixteenth-century apothecary put it, "It comes from choosing beds unknown and plugging holes best left alone."

Initially, surgeons tried to burn the poisonous humors out of the sores with hot irons, resulting in unspeakable pain and frequent infection. In his 1514 book *De Morbo Gallicus*, the Italian physician Giovanni de Vigo described a plaster he had invented made of mercury, lanolin, and olive oil to apply to the open genital sores of syphilis patients. The recipe proved so effective it remained in use in some form for nearly four hundred years.

Ambroise Paré often saw immediate results from mercury ointments. Muscle pain faded and the oozing sores dried up. "I my self have observed others," he wrote, "who thus, by the interposition of one or two daies, being rubbed over som fifteen or seventeen times, have perfectly recovered." Mercury ointments helped heal the ulcers by killing the *Treponema pallidum* bacteria that caused syphilis, though Renaissance doctors knew only that the treatments alleviated symptoms, as the bacteria wasn't discovered until 1905. But mercury, introduced into the bloodstream through the sores, could, over time, kill the patient, too.

Several times a day for up to thirty days, Ulrich von Hutten was smeared with quicksilver and other forms of mercury such as vermilion and cinnabar, along with rust from brass and iron, turpentine, hogs' lard, and powdered red worms. Ambroise Paré's recipe was a bit different: he mixed quicksilver with lead and boiled them in vinegar with sage, rosemary, thyme, chamomile, hogs' lard, turpentine, nutmegs, cloves, sage, lavender, marjoram, eggs, and sulfur, among other ingredients. The result must have been a lumpy, foul-smelling mud. Paré noted, "Regard must bee had of those parts, which are seazed upon by the symptoms of this diseas [the genital area], that they may bee more anointed, and that it may bee more thoroughly rubbed in."

Paré considered the treatment to be working when the patient spat and salivated excessively, what we now know to be a sign of mercury poisoning, but which he thought was the evacuation of evil humors.

A more aggressive treatment was to place the patient in a hot tent to inhale mercury, arsenic, antimony, and lead—four heavy metal poisons—mixed with turpentine and aloe. Mercury fumes went directly to the brain, causing brain damage. Hutten wrote, "Their Teeth fell out, and their Throats, their Lungs, with the Roofs of their Mouths, were full of Sores. Their Jaws did swell, their Teeth loosened, and a stinking Matter continually was voided from those places. Not only their lips, but the inside of their Cheeks, were grievously pained, and made the place where they were, stink most abominably, which sort of Cure was indeed so terrible that many chose rather to die than to be eased thus of their Sickness."

Hutten underwent this cure eleven times, "with great peril and jeopardy of Life, struggling with the Disease nine Years together, taking all the time whatever was thought proper to withstand the Disease, such as Baths with Herbs, Drinks and Corrosives." He was even given arsenic to drink, which, though it would have killed the syphilis bacteria, "occasioned such bitter pains that those might be thought very desirous of Life who had not rather die than thus to prolong it." During his "cures," Hutten saw several people die right in front of him when their throats swelled up and strangled them. One day he witnessed the physician pulling three men out of their mercury tent stone dead. Mercury treatment was, in a way, a sixteenth-century version of chemotherapy. If the horrible cure didn't kill you, it might even help you.

Paré, for one, realized the mercury inhalation cure was often worse than the disease. "I do not much approve hereof," he wrote, "by reason of sundrie malign symptoms which thence arise, for they infect and corrupt by their venomous contagion, the brain and lung, whence the patient dureing the residue of their lives have stinking breaths. Yea manie while they have been thus handled, have been taken hold of by a convulsion, and a trembling of their heads, hands, and legs, with a deafness, apoplexie, and lastly, miserable death." He added that through this treatment "manie have been brought into an uncureable consumption. In others sordid and putrid ulcers have thence arisen in the mouth, which having eaten a great part of the palate and tongue, have degenerated into a deadly Cancer." He also noted the excessive salivation after such a treatment. "For a whole moneth after," he wrote, "tough and filthie slaver hath continually flowed out of their mouths.

Other som have the muscles of their jaws relaxed; others troubled with a convulsion, so that dureing the rest of their lives they can scarce gape. Others by losing a portion of their jaw, have lost som of their teeth."

Even if the patient recovered completely after this torture, there was no guarantee that it would last. Syphilis could go into remission, but the bacteria never left the body before the advent of antibiotics in the 1940s. Paré added, "Ofttimes after ten years space, the diseas riseth as out of an ambush, or lurking-hole, and becomes far wors then before."

Because of the horrific side effects, when in 1529 the Italian jeweler to King François I of France, Benvenuto Cellini, contracted syphilis at the age of twenty-nine, he refused to undergo the mercury treatment. As the illness increasingly tormented him, Cellini, irascible at the best of times, now suffered from mood swings, megalomania, and paranoia. Some of his business partners, infuriated by his behavior, decided to kill him. They lured him to a dinner party and fed him a sauce laced with corrosive sublimate, a form of highly toxic mercury salt that was a favorite of Renaissance poisoners. Although Cellini suffered severe gastrointestinal symptoms and lay at death's door for days, the poison wasn't enough to kill him. It was enough, however, to send the *Treponema pallidum* packing. He rejoiced to find himself completely cured of syphilitic symptoms and lived another forty-two years.

One Italian royal, Isabella d'Aragona, who died in 1524 at the age of fifty-four, was not so fortunate with her mercury treatment for syphilis. When Dr. Gino Fornaciari of the University of Pisa exhumed her body from the Basilica di San Domenico Maggiore in Naples in 1984, he was immediately struck by her unusual teeth coated with a thick black patina, though in many places the black enamel had been abraded off, revealing white, if painful, surfaces below. The body voids mercury in the saliva, which turns teeth black. Some art historians believe that Isabella was the model for Leonardo da Vinci's *Mona Lisa*, and if so it's not surprising she has a pained, close-lipped smile.

Dr. Fornaciari also exhumed Isabella's brother, King Ferdinando II, who died in 1496 from a reported fever at the age of twenty-seven. Analysis of his remains revealed extraordinarily high levels of mercury in his hair as well as pieces of lice. Some of the mummies in the royal Neapolitan crypt had been treated with mercury as part of the embalming process, but only Ferdinando's hair showed high levels, an indication that he was using a mercury ointment to treat his lice infestation. Additionally, his bones were laden with extremely high levels of lead, either from medical treatments or from wine sweetened with lead, a common practice of the time.

By studying the corpses' hair, Dr. Fornaciari found that both Isabella and Ferdinando had been very sick for months before their deaths. Heavy metal toxicity disrupts the autonomous nervous system and metabolic rhythms, including hair growth. The normal growth rate of human hair is sixteen centimeters a year. Ferdinando's hair grew only twelve centimeters the year before his death, and Isabella's a shocking two centimeters. Years of chronic mercury poisoning eventually caused the irreversible collapse of Isabella's metabolism, called a "tipping point." Ferdinando was well on his way to tipping over himself from lead poisoning, but evidently a fever carried him away first.

CANNIBAL CURES

Human body parts, called *mumia*, were sold to apothecaries and physicians by the town executioner. Doctors believed that some essence of the life force remained in the body after death, especially in the case of executions or accidents where life was taken suddenly from an otherwise healthy young person. The remainder of the deceased's natural life span could thus be ingested by the person consuming his body parts.

According to Paracelsus, "The whole of the body is useful and good, and can be fashioned into the most valuable *mumia*. Although the spirit of life has gone forth from such a body, still the balsam remains, in which life is latent." However, a person who has died "a natural and predestined death," especially an older person, has used up his *mumia* and is of no value to the physician. "Let him be cast to the worms."

We know from court records that several monarchs—Charles II and William II of England, François I of France, and Christian IV of Denmark—were, in fact, cannibals when it came to their medicine. It is not known if Elizabeth I consumed body parts, but two of her favorite royal physicians heartily recommended it to their other patients. When James I of England suffered from gout (probably arthritis) starting in 1616, his physician, Théodore de Mayerne, recommended "an arthritic powder composed of scrapings of an unburied human skull, herbs, white wine, and whey, to be taken at full moon." But as "the king hates eating human bodies, an ox's head can be substituted in his case."

To cure epilepsy, doctors concocted recipes of dried human heart or made a potion of wine, lily, lavender, and an entire adult brain, which weighed about three pounds. Human fat was used to treat consumption, rheumatism, and gout. Physicians recommended those suffering from hemorrhoids to stroke them with the amputated hand of a dead man—a strangely unpalatable image to ponder.

Mummy flesh was venerated for its magical Egyptian antiquity and used for bruising, snakebites, and joint pain. King François I always carried some mummy flesh in his purse in case he fell and hurt himself. In 1703, the physician Robert Pitt wrote that "mummy had the honor to be worn in the bosom next [to] the heart by the kings and princes and all others who could then bear the price, in the last age, in all the courts of Europe."

In 1609, the German physician Oswald Croll stated in a recipe for a plague cure that one should "choose the carcass of a red [haired] man, whole, clear without blemish, of the age of twenty-four years, that hath been hanged, broke upon a wheel, or thrust-through [stabbed], having been for one day and night exposed to the open air, in a serene time." (We can only imagine how difficult it must have been to find exactly that . . . and in good weather.) The flesh should be cut into small slices and sprinkled with powder of myrrh and aloes before being repeatedly macerated in spirit of wine. After it has been "hung up to dry in the air," it would have a texture like smoked meat, a sign it was ready to be served.

Doctors believed that the vitality of a person who died of hanging or strangulation was forced up into the top of the skull at death. In the first part of the seventeenth century, Belgian chemist Jean Baptiste van Helmont explained that after death, "all the brain is consumed and dissolved in the skull," a kind of vitamin-rich intellectual stew. Charles II thought human skull was a basic cure-all and distilled it himself in his palace laboratory. However, even forty drops of it could not save him from his final illness.

In 1560, several Germans and Dutchmen working at the Royal Mint in the Tower of London fell suddenly ill, probably from exposure to copper fumes. The attending physicians believed that drinking from cups made from human skulls would cure them. Since no human skull cups were conveniently available, the rotting old heads of traitors adorning Tower Bridge were removed, the flesh boiled off, and the skulls fashioned into drinking vessels for the immigrant workers. Some of the men recovered, but most died despite their skull cups.

Human blood, too, was a cherished ingredient in medications. Doctors believed that vital spirits nestled within blood, and anyone drinking it would imbibe the life force itself. Dried and powdered blood was sprinkled on wounds or inhaled to staunch bleeding. The barber-surgeon who bled patients for a variety of ailments would turn around and sell their blood to others for use in medical recipes, thereby getting paid twice. Physicians recommended human blood for asthma, epilepsy, acute fevers, pleurisy, consumption, hysteria, convulsions, headaches, palsy, apoplexies, distempers, and jaundice, as well as in poison antidotes.

The patients most vulnerable to slipshod medical ministrations were new mothers. Many women, overjoyed at having survived the dangers of childbirth, were doomed to die horribly a few days later of puerperal fever. During and shortly after delivery, the uterus is a wide-open germ receptor. A physician sticking dirty hands or slimy instruments into a woman was unwittingly cultivating bacteria in a human petri dish, often resulting in a fatal case of sepsis.

Henry VIII's mother, Elizabeth of York, died of puerperal fever a few days after giving birth to a stillborn daughter in 1503. The same illness killed two of Henry's wives: Jane Seymour in 1537, after giving Henry his longed-for heir, the future Edward VI; and Henry's widow, Catherine Parr, who presented her fourth husband, Thomas Seymour, with a daughter in 1548. Catherine de Medici's mother, Madeleine de la Tour d'Avergne, most likely died of the same disease fifteen days after delivering Catherine in 1519.

No one knew the cause of puerperal fever until the 1840s when a young Hungarian doctor, Ignaz Semmelweis, noticed the horrifying mortality rate of new mothers at the Vienna General Hospital. Investigating the matter, he discovered that doctors often raced from the autopsy room—hands and instruments coated with stinking cadaver juice—to the delivery room and thrust them into the women in labor. Something in the corpse fluids was clearly harming the women.

Dr. Semmelweis instituted a strict sterilization routine for instruments and hands, which resulted in an immediate reduction of mortality from 18 percent to 3 percent. Other doctors, however, howled with protest. Semmelweis, they said, was not only wasting their time but was insulting them as gentlemen whose hands were always—metaphorically, at least—clean. Many in the medical profession heaped scorn and ridicule on Dr. Semmelweis, and the hospital where he had saved so many lives dismissed him. His rage at such unjust treatment consumed him. In 1865, at the age of forty-seven, he was placed in an insane asylum where, two weeks later, he died from a gangrenous wound caused by a severe beating by asylum guards.

In the 1880s, the German physician Robert Koch, a pioneering microbiologist, proved Semmelweis right: something in the corpse fluids had been killing the women, newly discovered germs that caused infectious disease. Semmelweis is now known as the father of antiseptic policy.

In rare cases, poisonous medications could send a patient stark, raving mad. In the summer of 1788, the plodding, fifty-year-old King George III of Great Britain began suffering painful stomachaches. He refused to take the doctors' medicines and improved quickly. But in October, he fell so ill he put himself wholly in their care. The doctors diagnosed an improper flow of bile. To correct the humoral imbalance, they gave him medicine to bring on projectile vomiting and diarrhea. They also blistered his scalp and applied leeches to his forehead to draw the evil humors out of his brain, and blistered his legs to pull the humors downward.

Within twenty-four hours of his first treatment, the king was feverish, his urine brown, his feet swollen, his eyeballs yellow, and his blisters festering and oozing pus. Even worse, his mental state deteriorated rapidly. He ran into a royal reception with his legs wrapped in flannel and babbled incoherently about losing the American colonies. During dinner, he slammed his eldest son violently against a wall. He spoke so quickly he could hardly breathe. He dictated orders to people who were long dead as foam bubbled out of his mouth. The medications left him vomiting, drenched in sweat, raving like a maniac, and howling like a dog. He danced the minuet with his servants and begged them to kill him. He thought that he was the emperor of Persia and that his pillow was his dead son. The king hated his medicines, but his doctors either forced him to take them—by trussing him up in a straitjacket chained to a chair until he did—or hid them in his bread and tea.

The king recovered in March 1789. But he suffered brief relapses in 1801 and 1805, during which the devoutly religious monarch tried to ride a horse into church and made the foulest suggestions to ladies of the court. In 1810, he was so devastated by the death of his favorite child, twenty-seven-year-old Princess Amelia, that he slipped once more into insanity and never fully recovered. Blind and mostly deaf, the king lived out his last years in Windsor Castle, often wearing mourning for himself as he believed he was dead, though he was rather happy about it. A month before his death at the age of eighty-one in 1820, he babbled nonstop for fifty-six hours.

Modern experts disagree about the nature of his illness. While some physicians argue that it was a purely psychological disease with some physical symptoms caused by his medications, others believe he had porphyria, a hereditary disorder resulting in abdominal pain, dark urine, weak limbs, hoarseness, excitability, paranoia, and schizophrenia, all of which the king suffered. Théodore de Mayerne, physician to George's great-great-great-great-grandfather, James I of England, wrote that the king had, among his many other ailments, urine "the color of Alicante wine," a deep red. Numerous descendants of Queen Victoria, George III's granddaughter, had lifelong health problems and periodic bouts of red or purple urine. In 1997, researchers exhumed Queen Victoria's granddaughter Princess Charlotte in Germany, scraped bone marrow from her leg, and found that she most likely had had the gene for porphyria. Queen Elizabeth II's first cousin, Prince William of Gloucester, was diagnosed with porphyria in 1968. Historians wonder whether the illness caused the bad health and strange mood swings of royals across Europe, from Mary, Queen of Scots in the sixteenth-century to her descendant Empress Alexandra of Russia in the early twentieth.

In 2003, a lock of George III's hair from the time of his death was found in a marked envelope in the basement of a London museum. While scientists were not able to extract DNA to test for the porphyria gene, they were able to conduct heavy metals analyses and determined that the hair contained over three hundred times the normal level of arsenic.

Some 90 percent of those who carry the porphyria gene have no symptoms whatsoever and never even know they have it. But attacks can be caused by alcohol, smoking, dieting, sunlight, and stress. One of the greatest triggers, however, is arsenic. Palace records indicate that throughout much of his life George used arsenic-based skin cream and wig powder. But during his periods of insanity, his doctors had him drink James's Powder, a compound of antimony laced with arsenic and prescribed for the reduction of fever, and Fowler's Solution, an arsenic-based tonic. It is unusual for the first symptoms of porphyria to show up when a carrier is fifty. Probably the king's attacks began only when the arsenic from his wigs and skin cream reached levels in his body high enough to trigger them. And, in an effort to cure the attacks, his doctors unwittingly gave him medicine that made them more violent and painful than before, eventually causing him to lose his mind completely.

More than two thousand years earlier, Alexander the Great succinctly summed up the situation on his Babylonian deathbed. "I am dying," the thirty-two-year-old lamented, "from the treatment of too many physicians."

5

PUTRID PALACES

A POISONED ENVIRONMENT

L ooking around our Ikea-filled apartments, many of us might utter a soul-deep sigh as we ponder the marble floors, gilt ceilings, and finely carved furniture of European palaces in centuries past. We would be less envious, perhaps, if we remembered that the most magnificent chambers were befouled by parasites, bacteria, viruses, and environmental poisons that carried far more victims to the grave than arsenic ever did.

Palaces were, in fact, a dominion of dung. Inside those lacquered cabinets were chamber pots brimming with a stinking stew of human waste. The contents of chamber pots were thrown down latrines, open holes with wooden seats and a straight shot down either into the castle moat, which frequently featured floating turds, or into the palace basement, which was only cleaned—and that must have been quite a job—when full to bursting. The human waste below Henry VIII's Great House of Easement, a two-story deluxe toilet facility at Hampton Court with twenty-eight holes, rose head-high before it was cleaned out.

Cesspits often burst through walls, either into the ground, leaching into groundwater and ending up in the nearest well, or into other rooms. On October 20, 1660, the London diarist Samuel Pepys had an unfortunate experience when the basement wall he shared with his neighbor was so saturated with human waste it leaked into his property. "When going down into my cellar," he wrote, "I stepped into a great heap of turds by which I found that Mr. Turners house of office [cesspit] is full and comes into my cellar, which do trouble me." No doubt it would trouble us all.

Those dazzling Baroque theaters, where Molière and Dryden debuted their witty plays, were also bursting with human waste. Each of the sumptuous private boxes had a chamber pot for its highborn guests. It strikes us somewhat odd, today, imagining friends and strangers blithely emptying their bladders and bowels beside us as we watch a performance. We can only hope they had the good manners to do their business behind a screen and, if the evacuation involved loud blasts, waited until the kettledrums and cymbals down in the orchestra drowned out the noise.

One evening in a Paris theater, according to Roger de Rabutin, comte de Bussy, two noblewomen—their names shall go down in eternal infamy as Madame de Saulx and Madame de Tremouille—each did a huge number two in their pot, "and then, to remove the evil smell, threw everything" onto the dismayed audience below, who shrieked their protest and chased the women out of the theater. Even by the lax standards of the seventeenth century that was going a bit far.

In large Spanish cities, authorities set up crosses in places used as latrines with the sign "Do not defecate where there are crosses." In the early seventeenth century, the poet Francisco de Quevedo wrote on the sign, "Do not put up crosses where I defecate."

Some courtiers even defecated in the public areas of the palace. A 1675 report on the Louvre in Paris claimed that "on the grand staircases . . . behind the doors and almost everywhere one sees there a mass of excrement, one smells a thousand unbearable stenches caused by calls of nature which everyone goes to do there every day."

Naturally, palaces offered numerous places to rid oneself of bodily waste, but when it came to urination, many male courtiers didn't go out of their way to use them, acting instead as if the world was their urinal. They did their business wherever the urge came upon them and assumed servants would clean up the mess they made. Stairwells, in particular, were popular urination points. (Some things never change.) Evidently some men even peed in the king's cooking hearth, as Henry VIII felt it necessary to issue an edict strictly forbidding it. They peed on garden walls, blending the joyous smell of roses with the rank smell of urine. Henry VIII instructed his servants to paint big red crosses on the walls as a deterrent to garden urinators, but it just gave them something to aim for.

A few months after Henry's death in 1547, the government of young Edward VI issued a proclamation forbidding anyone to "make water or cast any nuisance within the precinct of the court . . . wherein corruption may breed and tend to the prejudice of his royal person."

When the early sixteenth-century Dutch humanist Desiderius Erasmus wrote, "It is impolite to greet someone who is urinating or defecating," we can presume he was referring to a public place, and he felt the need to write this as it happened a lot. A 1570 German book of manners stated that "one should not like rustics relieve oneself without shame or reserve in front of ladies, or before the doors or windows of court chambers."

In 1518, when François I of France visited his mistress, the alluring twenty-three-year-old Françoise de Foix, dame de Châteaubriant, her secret lover, one Admiral Bonnivet, quickly jumped out of her bed and hid himself in her large fireplace. Luckily, it was summer and the hearth was filled with scented pine branches behind which Bonnivet concealed himself. Unluckily, the hearth also served as a latrine, and before making love to his mistress, the king unknowingly urinated on poor Bonnivet hiding under the boughs, soaking him to the skin, and in this uncomfortable and stinking position he had to remain all night listening to the sighs and grunts of his mistress having sex with the king.

The public heeding of nature's call was presumably the norm. When the Portuguese princess Catherine of Braganza, who had led a sheltered and pious existence, arrived in England to marry King Charles II in 1661, she and her ladies were shocked at finding men blithely urinating throughout the palace. They complained "that they cannot stir abroad without seeing in every corner great beastly English pricks battering against every wall." Louis XIV's no-nonsense German sister-in-law, Elizabeth Charlotte, wrote of Versailles Palace in 1702 that "the people stationed in the galleries in front of our room piss in all the corners. It is impossible to leave one's apartments without seeing somebody pissing." And in the early eighteenth century, the duc de Saint-Simon described an occasion when the Bishop of Noyon was overcome by such "a great desire to piss" as he passed the chapel of Versailles that he entered the upstairs section reserved for the royal family and peed over the balustrade, his urine bouncing off the consecrated floor of the church below.

While palace women usually had the good grace to relieve themselves in chamber pots, sometimes etiquette forbade it. During the reign of George I, one ill-starred lady-in-waiting to Caroline, Princess of Wales, feared her bladder would burst after attending her royal mistress for several hours in a palace drawing room. Forbidden by protocol from asking to be excused, the desperate woman spread her feet and peed on the floor, hoping no one would notice. Unfortunately, the resulting deluge spread across the polished tiles as wide as a dining table for ten, and almost inundated the princess's delicate satin slippers.

Until things got a bit cleaner in the eighteenth century, most royal courts traveled from one palace to another every two weeks or so. The Tudor court moved thirty times in a year. This frequent perambulation wasn't designed to enjoy the scenery, but to allow palaces to be scrubbed clean of urine and feces. The French court, too, was always on the move. In his autobiography, Benvenuto Cellini, a jeweler at the court of François I, wrote of eighteen thousand horses routinely ambling from one château to the next, along with hundreds of wagons crammed with royal furniture.

The glittering Palace of Versailles, in particular, was a challenge to keep clean. It was home to some several thousand courtiers and servants whose daily emissions of tons of bodily wastes had to go somewhere. But unlike most other royal residences, Versailles was not located next to a river that would sweep the foul stuff downstream. Chamber pots were dumped in carts or nearby cesspits that had to be cleaned out frequently. The situation was made worse in 1682 when Louis XIV decided to make it his permanent residence. Though he and a few friends might visit his palaces at nearby Marly or Saint-Cloud for cleaner air now and then, the court never entirely vacated Versailles. Scrubbing all that urine off the hearths, stairwells, and church floors had to be done hit or miss, and it was usually miss. Many physicians were perturbed not by the threat of infection from human waste—infection was not yet understood—but by its stinking fumes. Loathsome smells, they said, went right to the brain, turning it to mush.

While it was frowned upon for male servants to pee in corners and staircases, they were encouraged to do so in a vat in the kitchen so that their urine could be used as ammonia for cleaning the house as well as textiles such as draperies and clothing. In a rare protest against pee, in 1493 Parisian haberdashers appealed to the king himself to stop this practice because "bonnets cleansed by means of piss are neither proper nor appropriate nor healthful to place on one's head." Though the king agreed, by the 1540s the urine-using hat makers were back in business.

Even though soap was in use by the Middle Ages, some laundresses preferred to soak clothing in urine to eradicate the most stubborn stains. Because of its high ammonia content, really stale pee was used as a mordant, a substance that binds dye to cloth. The dyes of centuries ago—made from insects, barks, berries, roots, lichens, leaves, and flowers—would otherwise have faded quite easily.

Urea, a chemical compound naturally occurring in urine, was remarkably effective in softening and tanning animal hides. Book bindings, shoes, belts, saddles, and gloves were made from leather saturated with human urine. It was only in 1828 that the German chemist Friedrich Woehler discovered how to make urea from chemicals, thereby eliminating the need for pee-soaked clothing and leather.

THE HEALTH RISKS OF BATHING

It shouldn't surprise us that most people living in such filthy palaces were filthy themselves. And yet the educated Greeks and Romans of the Classical world—whom Renaissance kings and scholars worshipped— were scrupulously clean and bathed every day, sometimes soaking for hours while conducting business. Ancient doctors scrubbed their hands and instruments between patients. The ancients had no idea of germs or infection but simply thought filth was gross. Let us examine what happened in the intervening centuries that so completely changed ideas about dirt.

In the early fifth century, Rome's eleven aqueducts fed 1,212 public fountains and 926 public bathhouses. But in ad 537, invading Goths cut the aqueducts, making bathing much more problematic. The early

Catholic Church, which managed much of the day-to-day functioning of Rome in this tumultuous period, had no idea how to repair the aqueducts and declared that bathing should be curtailed anyway as it was a form of sinful hedonism practiced by pagans. A century later, this belief was further confirmed by a new sect of heathens—Muslims—who washed not once but five times a day, considered by the Christians to be clear evidence of their ungodliness.

A thick coating of dirt on the skin, the Church decreed, showed Christian humility and kept illness from entering the body. Over time, physicians came to believe that washing was dangerous, so dangerous, indeed, that many people consulted their astrologers to find the most auspicious time to take a bath. A popular sixteenth-century book, *This is the Myrour or Glasse of Helth*, advised, "Use not baths or stews, nor sweat too much, for all openeth the pores of a man's body and maketh the venomous air to enter and for to infect the blood."

In the late fifteenth century, Queen Isabella of Spain bragged that she had only bathed twice in her whole life. Queen Elizabeth bathed once a month, "whether she needed it or no," according to one contemporary chronicler. Her successor, James I, bore a great aversion to water and never bathed. One court lady complained that she and her friends got "lousy by sitting in a councillor's chamber that James frequented." King James didn't even wash his hands before eating. At table, he "only rubbed his fingers' ends slightly with the wet end of a napkin." His lover, the Duke of Buckingham, wrote in one letter to the king, "So, craving your blessing, I kiss your dirty hands." James itched constantly and rarely changed his clothes.

By contrast, in 1671, John Burbury, an English diplomat stationed in Istanbul, expressed his astonishment at the excessive "cleanliness of the Turks who, as they had occasion to make urine . . . afterwards washed their hands."

Over in France, Louis XIV had a similar dislike of personal hygiene. The Sun King frequently complained that his mistress, Madame de Montespan, wore too much perfume, which suffocated him. She turned a deaf ear because she doused herself not to hide her own body odor but his, as he apparently had bathed only twice in his life. In 1680, when the king accused his mistress of overweening pride and many other unworthy qualities, she replied scornfully "that if she had the imperfections of which he accused her, at any rate she did not smell worse than he." The ambassador from the wild, barbarous land of Russia—whose inhabitants indulged in the dangerous and bizarre habit of bathing regularly—agreed with the royal mistress, writing to the czar that Louis XIV "stank like a wild animal."

It may have been the king's lack of hygiene that, in 1685, caused an abscess to form in his anus, which by the following year had become a fistula, a narrow channel with one opening in the anal canal and the other in the skin near the anus. A fistula is often filled with pus and can be a starting point for a serious infection that spreads throughout the body. Not only were his evacuations excruciating, but the king couldn't ride, or walk, or even sit on his throne without great discomfort, giving new meaning to the term "a royal pain in the ass." A courageous barber-surgeon named Charles-François Felix agreed to operate, but only after experimenting on seventy-five human guinea pigs: "volunteers" from prisons, as well as men from the countryside who wanted to help the king. Not surprisingly, some of them died. Their sacrifice, however, was not in vain. Though the king had to be held down by four burly men, the operation was a complete success, and a grateful court proudly dubbed 1686 the Year of the Fistula. As everyone at court wanted to emulate the king, anal fistulas became all the rage at Versailles. Many courtiers claimed to have fistulas—a sudden source of pride. Male noblemen swaggering around the palace added a new accoutrement to their beribboned silk knee breeches: swathes of bandages elegantly draped over the rear end.

Even a century after the famous fistula, Versailles doctors still condemned the harmful effects of water, believing it to reduce one's energy and sex drive. Queen Marie Antoinette took a bath only once a month.

Washing the hair was considered downright dangerous, as evil humors were believed to more easily infiltrate a wet head than a dry one. A popular English proverb advised, "Wash they hands often, they feete seldom, and thy head never." In 1653, the English diarist John Evelyn resolved to wash his hair only once a year. Nobles would rub a cloth over their hair to remove the worst grease and dandruff or, if the physicians and astrologers concurred, wash it every few months in cold, herb-scented water.

In 1602, the Italian physician Bartolomeo Paschetti offered an excuse as to why ancient Greeks and Romans bathed so often and his own generation—which tried to emulate the Classical period in so many ways—did not. He wrote that bathing "was the discovery of the ancients for keeping the body fresh and clean, for since they did not have the custom of wearing linen garments . . . but in our own times since all, rich and poor alike, are accustomed to wear shirts and thereby more easily keep the body clean, the bath is neither so widely nor frequently employed as in the times of the ancients." While the linen shirts worn beneath doublets and gowns did absorb sweat, we must bear in mind that they were often worn day and night for days and even weeks at a time.

By the sixteenth century, the printing press churned out books that at least let literate people know they were being disgusting. Europe's first etiquette book, *Il Galatheo*, written in 1559 by Giovanni della Casa, disdained those "kinde of men that in coffing or neesing [sneezing], make suche noise, that they make a man deafe to here them, and spray upon all those nearby. Besides these there be some, that in yauning, braye and crye out like Asses." He was disgusted by those who dine "like swine with their snouts in the washe, all begroined, and never lift up their heads nor looke up, muche lesse kepe their hands from the meate, and with both their cheeks blowne, as if they should sound a trumpet or blowe the fier, not eate but ravon . . . Neither is it good maner, to rubbe your gresie fingers uppon the bread you must eat." The book stated that it was impolite to urinate in front of others, as well as to fart, belch, pick one's teeth, nose, or ears, or thrust a hand down one's breeches to scratch at fleas. "And when thou hast blowne thy nose," della Casa advised, "use not to open thy handkerchief, to glare uppon thy snot, as if thou hadst pearles and Rubies fallen from thy braynes."

SCRATCHING THE ROYAL ITCH

Living in such filthy palaces, and with infrequent recourse to washing, it is not surprising that royals and their courtiers were tormented by fleas and lice, many of which were brought into the palace by dogs. John Evelyn wrote that Charles II "took delight to have a number of little spaniels follow him and lie in his bed chamber, where often times he suffered the bitches to puppy and give suck." With their urine, turds, and fleas, these dogs rendered the room "very offensive and indeed made the whole Court nasty and stinking."

In the early seventeenth century, the great hall of Henry Hastings, the son of the fourth Earl of Huntingdon, was, according to a visitor, "strewn with marrow bones and swarmed with hawks, hounds, spaniels and terriers. From his wall hung the skins of recently killed foxes and polecats." Since heat-loving lice and fleas vacate their hosts once they are dead and cool, they would have dropped to the floor and hopped onto the humans and dogs passing by.

For centuries, little hyperactive dogs were used to turn a meat spit by the fire, and their fleas and lice jumped onto the kitchen workers and the food. Only in 1723 did the northern English landowner William Cotesworth order "the dog wheel to be moved in purpose to keep the dog from the fire, the wheel out of the way and the dog prevented from shitting upon anything it could." Even without the filthy little dogs, the boys who turned the spits in the hot kitchens could not help "interlarding their own grease to help the drippings," according to a Tudor report.

Until well into the seventeenth century, the floors of palaces and noble houses were covered with rushes, which hid from view the scraps of food people threw down, the urine of courtiers, and the turds of dogs. When the rushes grew rank, they were supposed to be replaced, but often fresh rushes were simply thrown on top of them. Filth such as this made royal palaces breeding grounds for insects, and no one was immune from them, not even kings. At the 1399 coronation of Henry IV of England, when the archbishop anointed the king's head with holy oil, lice rushed out of his hair, evidently angry about all the oil. And in 2008, Italian researchers examined the mummified remains of a fifteenth-century king of Naples, Ferdinando II of Aragon, and found lice in his head hair and pubic hair.

The advent of wigs helped curb such infestations. In 1655, the teenaged Louis XIV noticed that his hair was already receding and started the men's fashion of wearing huge curly wigs. His cousin Charles II followed suit when he became king of England in 1660. Suddenly wealthy men took to shaving their heads and wearing enormous poofy wigs, which offered a great advantage: lice, separated from the warmth and blood of their human host, die off in a day or two. They could not roost for very long in a wig.

Women—even those who wore wigs—didn't generally shave their heads, however. By the 1770s, they created towering coiffures that blended false hair with their own on wooden frames or padding, and coated the hair with grease to make the white powder stick. Such a creation took all day and was worn with minor touch-ups for at least a month. The woman whose scalp itched from the grease or lice would insert a head scratcher into the coiffure for relief.

Physicians of the time had no idea that parasite infestations were caused by filth and feces-contaminated drinking water. They thought that lice, worms, maggots, and fleas were spontaneously generated in human flesh. Medical experts also believed that sperm rotting inside a woman could mutate into worms. It wasn't until 1668 that the Italian physician and biologist Francesco Redi proved in his book *Experiments on the Generation of Insects*—considered a milestone in the history of modern science—that parasites came from outside the body. He conducted experiments in which he left some meat to rot out in the open on a table, upon which flies landed, while he set other meat under glass. After a few days, the meat rotting under glass had no insect infestations, while the open-air meat crawled with them. Still, most people laughed at him.

Worms were common among rich and poor alike. Excavations of latrine sites at the Louvre revealed that worms were rampant in the feces of court residents from the medieval period through that of Louis XIV. English King Richard III suffered intestinal worms that grew up to a foot long, as evidenced by the multiple roundworm eggs found on his pelvic bones.

In 2004, French researchers examined the remains of the fifteenth-century mistress of King Charles VII, Agnes Sorel, and found worm eggs mixed in with her bones, as well as the remains of plants used to eradicate them. She would have first swallowed roundworm eggs in food or drink contaminated with human feces. The tiny eggs would have migrated to her intestines to hatch, then swum through her bloodstream to her lungs. After maturing, the worms would have wandered up to the throat, where Agnes would have coughed some of them up—alive. Those that she swallowed would have returned to her intestines, mated, and hatched more eggs. Some of those would have been excreted in her waste, but others would have remained to continue the cycle.

In 1668, in Montpellier, France, a man voided a flatworm seven feet long. In 1655, a London innkeeper, Mr. Parry, desperately ill of a stomach ailment, voided in his chamber pot a total of twelve "serpents." Those who eagerly examined these serpents decided one had a head like a horse, another sported the head of a toad, and a third rather resembled a greyhound. After this astonishing evacuation, we can only assume Mr. Parry felt much better. In the mid-seventeenth century, when the sick and aging King Philip IV of Spain developed numerous boils, his physicians lanced them and were surprised to find bugs streaming out. Countless other people expelled strangely shaped creatures of all sizes from every orifice in their bodies. Autopsies revealed worms in the heart, liver, kidneys, and breasts. Sometimes they ate their way through the abdomen or popped out the navel.

Most physicians believed that fresh air was as dangerous as bathing, especially to the ill, young children, and pregnant women. Bedridden patients and women near their delivery were forced to live in a dark cocoon of smells from chamber pots, sweat, and sickness. A 2013 study of the skeletons of nine Medici children born in the sixteenth century revealed they all suffered from rickets, a vitamin D deficiency resulting in soft, misshapen bones. Six of the children had curved leg and arm bones, caused by trying to crawl or walk on extremely soft bones, and one of them had a deformed skull. Even short periods of time spent in sunlight trigger vitamin D production, but the grand ducal children, ranging in age from newborn to five years old, were probably swaddled inside the palace with little sunlight, a means of protecting them from the evil humors of fresh air.

In addition to keeping patients in dark smelly rooms, some doctors instructed sick people to lie on filthy sheets. The eminent seventeenth-century Dutch physician Ysbrand van Diemerbroeck advised those tending to smallpox victims to leave them in the same sheets for as long as two weeks. "Far better off it is to suffer the shifts of the patient, moist with sweat, to dry of themselves with the heat of the bed, and for the patient for some days to bear with the stench of the sweat, and the pustules coming forth, than to change his linen and be the cause of his own death." Freshly washed sheets were highly dangerous, according to the good doctor, because of the lethal smell of soap.

Henry VIII, arguably the cleanest monarch of his age, changed his body linen and sheets daily and bathed frequently. His sophisticated plumbing system at Hampton Court Palace brought piped water into the palace from conduit houses four miles away on a hill. Water was available in the king's bathroom, the kitchens, the Great House of Easement, the moat, and the fish ponds. Despite his unusual efforts to stay clean, even Henry VIII put pieces of fur in his bed in the hopes that vermin would jump onto the fur and not onto him.

TOXIC TOWNS

While many palaces and castles such as Versailles, Hampton Court, and Windsor were outside of teeming capitals, others—the Louvre, Whitehall, Florence's Palazzo Vecchio, and the Tower of London—were smack in the middle of extremely unhealthy conditions.

Residents of European capitals lived cheek by jowl in overcrowded houses. They dumped chamber pots into the streets below, and often onto the pedestrians. Cities crawled with fleas, lice, and rats. Knowing what we now do—that plague was caused by the bacterium *Yersinia pestis*, which was transmitted by bites from fleas carried on rats—we can well understand the frequent outbreaks across Europe. New studies have shown that the Black Death of 1348 wiped out at least half of Europe's population. For four centuries after that, the plague never truly left the continent, usually blossoming into a major epidemic and killing up to 30 percent of the population of a large city every generation or so. In 1466, 40,000 people died of plague in Paris. Venice lost 50,000 inhabitants in 1576–77 to plague, a third of the population. The outbreak of 1649 culled half of the population of Seville. In 1656, an epidemic killed half of Naples' 300,000 inhabitants. London's Great Plague of 1665 slaughtered 100,000 people, one out of every four residents.

Houses and palaces alike were perched on top of cesspits; roads were covered with human and animal waste; and well water could kill if not boiled or mixed with wine. In most major cities, river water was left in a bucket for several days so the solids could settle. Water from the top was scooped out and mixed with alcohol, which usually killed the germs. In 1778, Wolfgang Amadeus Mozart's mother, Anna Maria, chaperoning her son in Paris, died of dysentery from drinking the sewage juice known as Seine River water.

In 1853, cholera killed more than ten thousand people in London. A year later, a severe outbreak sickened thousands and killed 616 people in the Soho neighborhood in less than a month. Most authorities still believed epidemics were caused by excremental miasmas—unhealthful air seeping up from the ground. But Dr. John Snow investigated the outbreak and realized that most of the casualties had drunk water from a single public well, which had been dug only three feet from an old cesspit that we now know had begun to leak fecal bacteria. The contagion wasn't caused by foul air, Dr. Snow insisted, but by water contaminated by feces. Though the outbreak seemed to be coming to the end of its natural life cycle, he had the pump handle removed. The epidemic stopped and did not return. Still, members of London's Board of Health saw no correlation between fecal leakage, a public well, and cholera. Their report stated, "After careful inquiry, we see no reason to adopt this belief."

In 1883 the German bacteriologist Robert Koch published his work on the cholera-causing bacterium *Vibrio cholerae*, thereby proving Dr. Snow correct. Fortunately by then, London had already banished cholera due to the Great Stink of 1858. During a dry summer in which temperatures rose well over a hundred degrees Fahrenheit, the level of the Thames dropped precipitously, revealing banks covered with human waste. The entire city smelled like the inside of a very full chamber pot. Members of Parliament were so nauseated by the stench they soaked the riverside curtains of their chambers in lime chloride, to no avail. The chancellor of the exchequer, Benjamin Disraeli, called the river "a Stygian pool, reeking with ineffable and intolerable horrors." As a result, London's Metropolitan Board of Works constructed a comprehensive sewer system with eleven hundred miles of pipes.

Plague and cholera weren't the only diseases that ravaged everyone from beggars to monarchs. Typhoid fever, typhus, rotavirus, shigellosis, measles, diphtheria, whooping cough, bronchitis, pneumonia, smallpox, and tuberculosis were common. In 1509 Henry VII died of tuberculosis; his heir, Prince Arthur, had died in 1502 of tuberculosis or plague. In 1694 Queen Mary of England died of smallpox. In 1712, an epidemic—probably measles—swept through the Court of Versailles and killed Louis XIV's heir, his wife, and young son. Every suave courtier glittering with diamonds and rustling in silks was a potential Typhoid Mary, spreading infection to anyone they encountered.

But it wasn't only the living who spread sickness. Ever since the Black Plague of the 1340s, major European cities suffered from a surfeit of corpses. At the turn of the eighteenth century, the author Daniel Defoe witnessed the construction of expensive houses on top of plague pits from the 1665 epidemic that killed some one hundred thousand Londoners. "The houses . . . are built on the very same ground where the poor people are buried, and the bodies on opening the ground for the foundation were dug up, some of them remaining so plain to be seen, that the women's skulls were distinguished by their long hair, and of others, the flesh was not quite perished . . . and some suggested it might endanger a return of the contagion."

Cemeteries in major capitals overflowed—sometimes literally—with the dead. In Paris in 1780, after a month of heavy rain, the malodorous six-hundred-year-old Holy Innocents Cemetery in the heart of the city burst into the basement of a neighboring house. Grinning skeletons and rotten coffins piled up to the ceiling, to the shock and horror of the homeowner standing agape on his basement steps holding up a lantern. Louis XVI ordered the bones of all Parisian cemeteries to be transported to catacombs beneath the city or places outside the walls. Over a period of twelve years, some six million bodies were moved.

It took sixty years for London politicians to follow suit. London was chock full of graveyards. Each church had one, and others were wedged in between shops, houses, and inns and next to wells and pumps. Over time, millions of bodies had been packed on top of one another. To earn a quick profit, cemetery owners hacked up coffins after a few days, threw quicklime on the bodies, and squeezed in more burials. In 1839, the London physician and public health activist George Walker (known as Graveyard Walker for his habitual perambulations around city cemeteries) described a church on a major thoroughfare. "The ground is so densely crowded as to present one entire mass of human bones and putrefaction which are in the course of further interments exhumed by the shovelfuls." He added, "The soil of this ground is saturated, absolutely saturated, with human putrescence."

Exposure to toxic gases exuded by corpses—methane, hydrogen sulfide, and the aptly named cadaverine and putrescine—can be fatal. In one such case in 1838, Thomas Oakes, the gravedigger of London's Aldgate Church, collapsed and died at the bottom of a pit grave containing numerous bodies thrown in without coffins. A heroic young man named Edward Luddett grabbed a ladder, climbed down to help, and "the instant he stopped to raise the head of Oakes, he appeared as if struck with a cannon ball, and fell back . . . and appeared instantly to expire."

Because gas from corpse pits could kill those in the immediate vicinity, physicians of the time believed that corpse-generated illnesses were transmitted via the air, when they were, in fact, carried in the water. Many churchyards had wells in their courtyards to serve the local community. London's St. Clement Church had a pump located just a few feet away from graves, but in 1807, according to one eyewitness, the water "had become so offensive, both to the smell and the taste, that it could not be used by the inhabitants, owing, most probably, to the infiltration of the dissolved products of human putrefaction."

By the 1860s, most of the London cemeteries were closed, and the bodies removed and re-interred in new garden cemeteries outside the city, such as Highgate.

THE ADVERSITIES OF ALCHEMY

As if the feces, urine, germs, and dead bodies weren't enough of a health threat, many gentlemen scientists set up complex alchemical laboratories in their homes that spewed mercury, lead, and other poisons into the very air they breathed. Alchemy was the search for the legendary philosopher's stone, a substance capable of turning lead, mercury, or other base metals into gold. By 1720, alchemy was discredited as the domain of fools and charlatans, though chemistry—with its strict scientific protocols—owes a debt of gratitude to alchemy for its very existence. Alchemists discovered the basic principles of chemistry.

One English king's love for pottering around in his alchemy lab killed him, according to a recent report. Charles II, always short of money with his expensive mistresses and even more expensive wars, hoped to find the solution to his financial woes by turning base metal into gold. He had a lab built in the basement of Whitehall Palace where he frequently conducted experiments. The diarist Samuel Pepys took a tour; he described it as a "pretty place" in which he saw "a great many Chymicall glasses and things, but understood none of them."

Charles and his assistants worked primarily with mercury ore and quicksilver, heating them in huge vats to combine with other substances. Given the complete lack of safety precautions in a seventeenth-century lab, Charles would have inhaled odorless mercury vapor on a regular basis. In 1967, the University of Glasgow examined a lock of his hair using neutron activation analysis techniques and found mercury ten times higher than normal. The king showed symptoms of chronic mercury poisoning in his behavior, as well. Renowned for his happy-go-lucky temperament, by 1684 he suffered mood swings, irritability, and depression. Courtiers thought the fifty-four-year-old king was just getting old and cranky. Then, on February 2, 1685, there was likely an explosion in the lab, exposing Charles to a lethal amount of the poison, which he inhaled without even being aware of it.

When Charles got up in the morning to use the chamber pot, he tried to speak but could not. "It was perceived by those in his chamber that he faltered somewhat in his speech," according to a witness. After visiting his closet, "he was taken with a fit of apoplexy and convulsions." He suffered three more convulsive fits and symptoms similar to those of a stroke, which rendered him speechless for a time.

The next torture was administered by his twelve doctors, who over the following days endeavored by various means to draw out the evil humors causing his condition. They removed sixteen ounces of blood at a time, shaved his head, and applied a blistering agent and red-hot irons to his scalp. Then they put caustic plasters on the soles of his feet to raise blisters. The learned physicians prepared potions for him that induced violent vomiting and a steady stream of diarrhea. They gave Charles a drink with Spanish fly, also known as cantharides, an irritant that causes topical blistering. But when it is consumed, cantharides weakens the kidneys and causes burning urination and sometimes death. To prevent him from biting his tongue during his convulsions, they jammed a stick into his mouth, which wounded his throat. Then they took ten ounces of blood from his jugular vein. They fed him extract of human skull and the magical bezoar stone. As he slipped into unconsciousness, they took another twelve ounces of blood. He died four days after the onset of symptoms, shortly before noon on Friday, February 6.

The physicians who performed the autopsy were perplexed by the appalling state of the king's brain. This was no ordinary stroke; in fact, he had never been paralyzed and had completely regained the power of speech after a brief interval. The autopsy revealed that while all his other organs were normal, and the brain had no bleeding, swelling, or tumor, the usually crystal-clear fluid surrounding the brain was swimming in serum—the protein-containing part of the blood—which we now know means that the blood-brain barrier had been breached.

In his 2003 book, *The Sickly Stuarts*, Frederick Holmes, professor emeritus of the University of Kansas Medical Center, wrote that the only possible explanation for the breach is that the king inhaled a large amount of mercury vapor at one time. Mercury is one of the few substances that can cross the blood-brain barrier, which protects against toxins. Minor doses of inhaled mercury cause no immediate symptoms, but a sizable serving of the poison would have gone from the king's lungs directly to his brain, where it vitiated the cells, causing Charles's strokelike symptoms. Whatever minuscule chance he may have had to recuperate from such a serious brain injury was vanquished by his doctors' murderous efforts to cure him.

A few years later, Sir Isaac Newton, the father of modern physics, almost suffered the same fate as King Charles. Newton, too, experimented with mercury, lead, arsenic, and antimony, though not in a get-rich-quick scheme: he wanted to understand the chemical processes involved in transmuting one substance into another. He cooked them over an open flame, inhaling the vapors. "After I had stirred the mercury and salt together," he wrote in his diary, "I put it on the fire to evaporate. The salt flew away quickly and left the mercury congealed in a hard rugged lump." Newton even tasted the toxin, calling it "strong, sourish ungrateful." Newton increased his mercury exposure by painting most of his walls red; the color was created using vermilion, a mercury-rich pigment.

Always eccentric, in 1693, at the age of fifty, Newton became a recluse, telling all his friends he never wanted to see them again for various imagined persecutions. Newton suffered paranoia, memory loss, insomnia, and lack of appetite—all symptoms of mercury poisoning.

In 1979, neutron activation and atomic absorption analysis of a lock of Newton's hair, thought to have been cut at the time of his death in 1727, found that he had about four times more lead, arsenic, and antimony than normal, and fifteen times more mercury. We can only speculate that the levels in his hair back in 1693 would have been far higher.

Unlike poor King Charles, who evidently suffered a fatal blast of mercury playing with his chemistry set, Newton survived his long-term, low-grade poisoning, perhaps by putting away his toxic cookpots and concentrating on optics, calculus, astronomy, and several other non-lethal areas of interest. After only six months of illness, he regained his usual temperament—which was only marginally better than his poisoned one—and lived to be eighty-four.

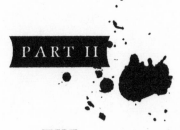

PART II

THE

Poison Chronicles

WHERE RUMORS *of* ROYAL POISONING
MEET SCIENTIFIC ANALYSIS

NATURAL ILLNESS, ACCIDENTAL POISONING, OR MURDER?

Numerous royals, important nobles, and court artists have reportedly been poisoned over the centuries. But were the vomit-spewing, sheet-soiling illnesses the result of arsenic, or toxic cosmetics, medications, and surroundings? Let's examine the stories of twenty palace personages who were reputedly poisoned, as well as their final illnesses, contemporary autopsies, and modern analyses of the bodies or hair, if available.

Even without remains of any kind, it is possible for researchers today to identify a probable cause of death if there are detailed reports of the final illness and an autopsy. By the Renaissance, doctors kept copious notes of royal illnesses—probably because they didn't want to be accused of ineptitude or intentional murder—with details of fever and other symptoms, as well as the medical treatments they administered. The results of autopsies, too, were carefully recorded. With these reports, today's physicians can speculate whether poison or natural causes carried off the deceased, and if the death was natural, the particular ailment involved.

Modern technology such as mass spectrometry and neutron activation analysis can detect the presence of poisons in human remains and, based on their levels, help us guess as to whether the poison was a toxic dose intended to kill or a remedy used to cure or beautify. In four intriguing cases, it seems that physicians intentionally gave their patients not a healing balm, but death in a cup.

6

HENRY VII of LUXEMBOURG,
HOLY ROMAN EMPEROR, 1275–1313

On August 8, 1313, in the stifling heat of an Italian summer, the thirty-eight-year-old Holy Roman emperor, Henry VII of Luxembourg, marched south from Pisa with his massive army. The emperor's enemies trembled at what was coming: pitched battles, besieged cities, burned crops, fire, rape, murder, conquest. Sixteen days later and only sixty-eight miles into his journey, the emperor was dead, poisoned in his communion wine, it was said. And in 2013, Italian researchers analyzing the body indeed found copious evidence of poison—but not from communion wine.

In 1308, German bishops and princes elected Henry, the ruler of a minor duchy wedged between Germany and France, as the new King of the Romans and emperor-elect of the Holy Roman Empire. He would only become emperor after his coronation in Rome. The new monarch was eager to head south and be crowned, unaware that the title was more glitter than gold.

More than three centuries after the fall of the Roman Empire, Charlemagne had revived the title of emperor in ad 800, and it would limp along for a thousand years until Napoleon put it out of its misery in 1806. The renowned eighteenth-century French philosopher François-Marie Arouet—known by his *nom de plume*, Voltaire—famously stated,

"The Holy Roman Empire is neither holy, nor Roman, nor an empire." He was right.

What was it, then? An anachronism. A battered crown plucked from the wreckage of lost dreams. A loosely organized political alliance of squabbling territories, with the emperor playing the role of an exasperated school principal disciplining unruly children bearing swords. Yet the title had a seductive allure that few could resist, despite the constant conflict in the emperor's Italian domains.

In Italy in the eleventh century, the friction between popes and Holy Roman emperors had flared into civil war. Guelphs supported the pope—God's spiritual vicar—and Ghibellines the emperor—God's temporal vicar. In a fascinating bit of historical trivia, Napoleon owed his surname to the conflict. In the twelfth century, his Florentine ancestors called themselves Buonaparte—the good party—because they were Ghibellines. As with most religious conflicts, the Guelph-Ghibelline struggle had nothing to do with God and everything to do with power and greed. Warlords used it as an excuse to invade, steal, and pillage. It was, in actuality, nothing more than a centuries-long grab fest.

Though no emperor-elect had been to Italy for sixty years, Henry, an idealist, leaped at the opportunity to bring peace to the war-torn peninsula. Known for his kindness and temperate manner of living—unlike most medieval rulers—he administered his little kingdom of Luxembourg efficiently and fairly. He would now dispense justice on a far grander scale, he vowed, forcing Italian municipalities to compromise, negotiate, and, under his beneficent rule, live peacefully. He would outlaw the very mention of the names Guelph and Ghibelline, causing all to live as loving Christians in a new golden age.

When Henry first arrived in Lombardy, in north Italy, his new subjects were impressed with his good looks. Clean-shaven and slender, with short red hair, the emperor-elect had a pink complexion, arched eyebrows, and a pointed nose and chin. They were less impressed by his political edicts: revamping governments, forcing cities to take back political exiles, opening jails, returning confiscated property, and imposing heavy taxes to support his court and army. Though Henry strove to show political impartiality, he had as little understanding of the complexity of Italian affairs as he did of the Italian language, and spoke only French and Latin.

While some war-weary Italians such as Dante Alighieri hailed the arrival of this justice-loving, chivalrous ruler as "the king of peace," many others were horrified by an emperor who really wanted to rule. A glittering coronation followed by a raucous party was one thing they could get behind, but they found the bungling intrusions of this dreamy-eyed northern invader quite obnoxious.

Henry was soon drawn into contentious local quarrels and forced to take sides. Enemies lined up against him. Many cities refused to pay their imperial taxes, or let him change their laws, or welcome back trouble-making political opponents. His greatest enemy was King Robert of Naples, the pope's champion who harbored his own expansionist dreams and wanted no competition from this simpleminded interloper.

When Henry entered Rome for his coronation in June 1312, he found that Guelph troops led by King Robert's brother barred the way to St. Peter's. After a fierce street-by-street battle in which he lost many men, he gave up on St. Peter's and was crowned in the church of St. John Lateran as Emperor Henry VII. The coronation banquet was interrupted by rocks raining in through the windows as guests ducked under tables.

The prosperous Guelph Republic of Florence was the most outspoken opponent of imperial supremacy. In August 1312, the ruling Florentine body, the *Signoria*, wrote to King Robert, "If that enemy [Henry] should be killed, as might easily occur, there is no doubt that in the future no disturber of you or us will rise up in the name of the Empire or will dare or presume to come to your lands or ours." It remains unclear whether the Florentines were thinking that Henry might die in battle or from natural illness or if this was a veiled plan to murder him.

Frustrated and outraged, the emperor dropped his platitudes of peace and forgiveness and waged war in earnest against his ungrateful enemies. He spent the spring and summer of 1313 in Pisa assembling a huge army and an imperial fleet. Despite feeling unwell, on August 8, he ignored his physicians' advice and set out with his forces to vanquish King Robert. Henry would march to Rome first and, having conquered the city, sail to Robert's kingdom in Sicily.

Though reports of his march are vague and sometimes contradictory, it seems that the army's progress was unusually slow because Henry stopped at various thermal baths in the area in the hopes of healing his fever and an abscess on his hip. He had first become ill two years earlier when besieging the town of Brescia. According to a contemporary chronicler, "The air was corrupted by the stink of horses . . . and many of the northerners became sick, and many great barons died, and they left due to illness and then died on the road."

The illness? Anthrax, most likely. Until the turn of the twentieth century, anthrax was as much a plague among humans as it was animals. Even those residents of the most sophisticated cities, such as Paris and Rome, lived side by side with anthrax-bearing horses, cows, sheep, pigs, and goats. Anthrax can be transmitted by eating, inhaling, or touching the spores of an infected animal, though it is rarely transmitted from human to human. Horrifyingly, anthrax spores in a buried carcass are still infectious centuries later.

Intestinal anthrax causes nausea, abdominal pain, intestinal lesions, bloody vomiting and diarrhea, and, in Henry's day, would have had close to a 100 percent mortality rate. Inhalational anthrax, too, would almost always have been fatal; it causes fever, chest pain, and pneumonia. Skin anthrax causes painless black sores that resemble cigarette burns and give off a nauseating stench, which would explain "the stink of horses" in the Brescia epidemic. It has the lowest rate of death, about 20 percent if not treated with modern medicine. At the siege of Brescia, the hundreds of dead horses would have been buried in deep grave pits to prevent further contagion. Humans maneuvering horse corpses and inhaling the stench would have become infected. It is possible the anthrax infected not only horses, but spread to the cows, pigs, and goats in the camp, and was consumed by soldiers in meat cooked unevenly over an open campfire.

Henry's army took the illness with them as they limped north. His queen, Margaret of Brabant, died of an epidemic that contemporaries called "plague" in Genoa in December 1311. A year later, while Henry's troops were encamped around Florence, another epidemic—perhaps the same kind—struck. According to the bishop of Butrinto, "A great illness and mortality began in the camp . . . which corrupted the district up to Florence." The physicians "despaired about the emperor."

Now, in August 1313, Henry tried to ignore his alarming symptoms and continue his march south. While camping near Siena, according to the Paduan statesman and historian Albertino Mussato, the emperor "felt come over him a kind of languor and went to bed before his usual hour, but laying down on the bed he could not sleep. However, upon waking, there was a pustule on a leg, beneath his right knee, and tormented by pain that it gave him, spent the night without sleep." The following dawn, he insisted the army pull up camp and march to the town of Buonconvento, twelve miles away, where he became so ill he could march no further.

After three days of extremely high fever, Emperor Henry VII, would-be savior of Italy, died. Within a few days, his armies dispersed. As the imperial corpse lay cooling, Henry's attendants decided that he had been killed by poisoned communion wine, which was never tested by a taster but handed directly from priest to communicant. The rumor mill even identified the poisoner, a Dominican priest in his sixties named Bernardino de Montepulciano who was probably Henry's confessor and who, hearing the rumors, wisely disappeared after the emperor's death. Northern Europeans eagerly accepted the story of a treacherous Italian killing their beloved emperor. The annals of the German monastery of Luttlich recorded that the emperor "was killed by poison in the Sacrament of the Mass." The Benedictine monastery at Freising affirmed, "He hoped to take the cup of salvation but took the cup of death."

But the contemporary Italian historian Tolomeo da Lucca, also a Dominican, had a different story. "In the month of August," he wrote, "the emperor was in the area of Siena near Buonconvento and became sick. He died a natural death . . . although some evil-minded people said he had been given poison in his Eucharist."

The priest had supposedly murdered Henry on the orders of Pope Clement V. Or Robert of Naples. Or the Republic of Florence. There were so many people who wanted Henry and his army gone from Italian soil that there was an embarrassment of choices. Much of Italy actually celebrated the emperor's demise. According to a Sienese chronicler, as soon as the Guelphs learned the news, "The Florentines, Sienese, Luchese and Pistoians and those bound to them had great joyfulness." In the city of Parma, according to a contemporary chronicler, "The bells did not cease pealing for joy. And such festivities lasted for eight days and more."

A historian hearing of a feverish death in an Italian August would automatically think of malaria. But malaria does not cause abscesses or pustules. It is likely that Henry's black anthrax lesions became infected and suddenly weren't the painless kind anymore. Red, hot, swollen lesions would have sent toxemia through his bloodstream, causing a fever and, after several days, killing him.

Albertino Mussato wrote, "It was verified that there were three causes of his death: first, the fatal ulceration below his knee that was called anthrax by the doctors; second, a broken bladder as a result of a slow and painful discharge of urine, with which he usually showed great patience; third, pleurisy [inflammation of the lining of the lungs]." The bladder and lung infections could have been separate issues from the anthrax, or could have been part of a massive infection spreading through the emperor's body caused by anthrax-induced toxemia.

On his deathbed, Henry had indicated that he wanted to be buried in Pisa. His devastated attendants duly carted his body northward, but his corpse, melting in the August heat and riddled with anthrax lesions, gave off such a foul smell they couldn't continue. They subjected the remains to a method devised to bring back the remains of German crusaders from the Holy Land without the coffins exploding from decomposition gases: they cut off his head, boiled the entire body, scraped off the skin and muscles, and burned the batch of bones.

A more cheerful group of mourners then took these nonoffending remains to Pisa. Henry was interred in the cathedral in 1315 after his magnificent tomb was completed.

MODERN POSTMORTEM AND DIAGNOSIS

As part of the ceremonies around the seven-hundredth anniversary of Henry's death, in 2013 researchers from the University of Pisa opened his tomb. Inside they found a crown, scepter, and orb, all made of gilded silver. Wrapping the bones was a magnificent silk cloth ten feet long and four feet wide of faded blue and red stripes with gold- and silver-embroidered lions.

The analysis of Henry's charred bones revealed he had been about five foot nine and well built. His left forearm showed signs of stress from a repetitive motion such as holding a bridle or weapon. His muscles had been more developed below the waist than above, and his legs a bit bowlegged. Clearly, this man had spent a great deal of time in the saddle. His knees showed signs of long periods of kneeling; we can assume it was in prayer. Scientists also found high levels of arsenic in his bones, though this could not have been caused by poisoned communion wine. If the priest had given the emperor a toxic spoonful of arsenic in the blood of Christ, it wouldn't have had time to make it to his bones. It would have shown up in his liver and stomach, which were boiled and scraped away soon after. The fact that the arsenic was in his bones indicates that he had been absorbing it over a period of weeks or even months.

How did the arsenic get in Henry's bones? The answer is simple. For centuries, physicians used it as a remedy against anthrax, mixing grains of arsenic with mercury and rubbing the ointment on the open lesions. Extremely high levels of mercury were also found in Henry's bones. Medical practitioners knew, of course, that arsenic was poisonous. But through trial and error they had found that in small amounts it could heal skin conditions such as anthrax lesions. What medieval physicians didn't know was the reason it worked: arsenic killed bacteria, just as in larger amounts it killed humans. While prescribing such a dangerous treatment, physicians advised the patient to eat a great deal of flour and other cereals, which they believed would diminish the medication's harmful effects. Researchers discovered large amounts of magnesium, found in flour and cereals, in Henry's remains.

Henry died of a fever. But over the course of months, or perhaps even two years, the chronic poisoning surely would have weakened him, allowing the anthrax to tip him over the edge more easily.

7

CANGRANDE della SCALA, ITALIAN WARLORD, 1291–1329

On July 18, 1329, Cangrande della Scala, the thirty-eight-year-old warlord of Verona, rode triumphantly into the city of Treviso on a magnificent white horse to celebrate his conquest. After more than twenty years of warfare, his life's ambition of ruling a swath of northern Italy had finally been achieved. But within four days, the strapping warrior would be dead, and in 2016 scientists would find the most astonishing substance in his mummified rectum.

Cangrande was the son of Alberto I della Scala, lord of Verona. Originally christened Can Francesco, over time his loyalty and courage earned him the name of Cangrande—the Great Dog. In the centuries-long wars of the Guelphs and Ghibellines, the Scaligeri, as the family was known, were firmly Ghibelline and enthusiastically supported the new Holy Roman emperor, Henry VII of Luxembourg. Henry rewarded Cangrande by making him lord of Vicenza in 1312. After the emperor's death the following year, Cangrande continued to fight Guelph cities for his own aggrandizement.

Cangrande was one of the finest warriors in Europe. He showed jaw-dropping bravery on the field of battle, as well as the ability to inspire similar feats of heroism among his men. He plucked arrows out of his wounds and continued fighting. He was the first to scale castle walls.

If defenders pushed his ladder over and he toppled into the moat, he dragged himself out and climbed back up. Albertino Mussato, a historian fighting with the Paduan army, wrote that Cangrande stood up in his stirrups, commanded his men to "slay the cowardly foe," and raced forward swinging his mace right and left, carrying all before him "as fire fanned by the wind devours stubble."

But Cangrande was no mere brutish berserker. He possessed the cultivated qualities so prized in the burgeoning Italian Renaissance. He was generous to fallen enemies, gallant with the ladies (he sired at least eight bastards, a fact applauded by most Italians), a brilliant conversationalist, an inspirational orator, a wily politician, and a lover of poetry, art, and literature. Wildly charismatic and in love with life, he was known for the rare beauty of his smile and a charm that mesmerized friend and foe alike.

Cangrande welcomed countless exiles from other cities and hosted them at his own table for years on end. Among them were nobles, poets, and scholars, including Dante Alighieri, who had been expelled from his native Florence for ending up on the wrong side of the political divide and lived as Cangrande's guest at various times between 1312 and 1318. In short, the court of Verona was renowned as the grandest and most cultured in all Italy.

Even Cangrande's monstrous arrogance and periodic temper tantrums were seen as strengths in a medieval Italian warlord. Perhaps most unusual for one in his position, instead of stuffing his pockets with riches stolen from his people, he taxed them fairly and administered justice wisely. Cangrande became known as the living manifestation of chivalrous knighthood.

After trying for seventeen years to capture the rich city of Padua, in 1328 he was invited by the city to take it over and end violent civil unrest. Now, with three cities in his belt, there was only one more he longed to conquer: Treviso. In early July 1329, Cangrande's army besieged the city. On July 17, Treviso surrendered. After two decades of warfare, Cangrande was now master of a wide and prosperous region and boasted four shining jewels in his crown: Verona, Vicenza, Padua, and Treviso. His dream had come true. But it was not to last.

When, on July 18, he made his state entry into Treviso, he wasn't feeling well. A few days earlier, on the march from Padua, he had drunk

cold water from a "polluted" spring, according to contemporary accounts, which gave him a fever, vomiting, and diarrhea. Most likely, the
pollution referred to soldiers' excrement. After his victorious ride
through town, he slid off his horse at the bishop's palace where he would
lodge and took to his bed. He managed to deal with various items of
business until the afternoon of July 20, when he realized he might not
survive and made his will. Two days later, he was dead. With no
children by the woman he had married when he was seventeen, his neph-
ews, twenty-two-year-old Alberto and twenty-year-old Mastino della
Scala, took over his dominions.

Naturally, rumors of poison flew around Italy, and according to the
Paduan ambassador to Verona at the time, Mastino had one of Cangrande's doctors hanged for the death of his uncle, though whether it
was for murder or negligence we do not know. For centuries, historians
have wondered what killed the conqueror. Dysentery from the polluted
spring? A burst appendix? A perforated ulcer? Or poison? Nearly
seven hundred years after Cangrande's death, the answer has been
revealed.

MODERN POSTMORTEM AND DIAGNOSIS

In February 2004, a team of Italian researchers from the University of
Pisa cracked open Cangrande's ornate tomb at the church of Santa
Maria Antica in Verona to confirm or refute the rumor of arsenic poisoning. They were shocked to see the condition of the body: no sad
heap of rotten bones, but a natural mummy with intact flesh and remarkably preserved organs, a great boon for determining whether he
had died of natural illness or poison. Even the mummy's striped Ori-
ental robe remained in a decent state of preservation.

The five-foot-seven-inch corpse lay on its back with its arms folded
across the chest. Researchers took digital X-ray and CT scans, as well as
samples from the hair, liver, and feces in the rectum. They found that
Cangrande suffered from a mild form of black lung disease and emphy-
sema, probably from huddling around all those campfires on campaign.
He also had some arthritis in the elbows and hips, evidence of years in
the saddle. Gold and silver levels were quite high in his hair, most
likely due to the burial cloth embroidered with gold and silver thread
that had covered his head. But he also had high levels of gold, silver,

and lead in his liver tissues from a lifetime of exposure to clothing as well as eating and drinking utensils made from these substances. Which brings us to a sobering conclusion: while most of us would like to have been born with a silver spoon in our mouths, it could have been hazardous to our health.

Researchers found that Cangrande had thrown up immediately before he died, as regurgitated food thickly coated his esophagus. In his digestive tract, they discovered chamomile pollen, black mulberry, and lower-than-average arsenic levels; thus, the rumor that Cangrande died of arsenic poisoning was patently false. But the team did find lethal amounts of poison in the form of digitalis, the foxglove plant, which also showed in the liver. Given that much of the toxicity would have leached out over the past seven hundred years, he must have consumed an extraordinary amount of the stuff.

Eating any part of the foxglove plant—the roots, flowers, or leaves—causes nausea, vomiting, diarrhea, hallucinations, vision disturbances, and a change in heart rate than can result in heart block, or interference with the heart's electrical signals that keep it pumping. Large amounts can so confuse the heart that it simply stops. Cangrande's symptoms—other than the fever—were consistent with digitalis poisoning. But digitalis does not cause fever.

It seems that he started off with a natural illness, one quite common for an army on the march and one that he probably had had before and would have survived again this time. Then his physician gave him a medicinal preparation for his illness, as evidenced by chamomile, used as a sedative and to combat fever, and black mulberry, used to disguise the sour tastes of medicine with its sweetness. But mixed in with the helpful ingredients was a fatal dose of digitalis, which would have increased the diarrhea and vomiting and, in such huge amounts, ultimately stopped his heart.

How did the digitalis get in the medicinal preparation? Medical and botanical writings from the Roman Empire on describe foxglove as poisonous to consume. It was only used topically to treat sprains, bruises, and snakebites until the late eighteenth century, when it was discovered that consuming tiny amounts could treat heart conditions, water retention due to kidney disease, and epilepsy. In the late nineteenth century, Vincent van Gogh's doctor may have prescribed digitalis for the artist's epilepsy, which would have caused him to see stars with huge yellow halos around them, forming the theme for his *Starry Night*. Even then, it was prescribed reluctantly due to the difficulty in distinguishing between a therapeutic dose and a dangerous one.

It is possible that when Cangrande took to his bed immediately after his triumphal entry into Treviso, one of his enemies paid his doctor to poison him. Neighboring powers such as the duchy of Milan or the Republic of Venice probably felt threatened by his expanding influence. Or the murderer could have had more personal reasons. Perhaps Mastino, Cangrande's ambitious nephew and one of his heirs, could have done it.

On the other hand, could the doctor—in his desperation at possibly losing such a powerful patient—have grabbed the wrong leaves from his bag of herbs?

And so we see that even when some mysteries are solved, new ones take their place.

8

AGNES SOREL, MISTRESS of KING
CHARLES VII of FRANCE, 1422–1450

On a cold winter's day, twenty-eight-year-old Agnes Sorel, the most beautiful woman in France, lay dying in the tidy stone manor house of the Abbey of Jumièges, some eighty miles northwest of Paris. She often traveled there to give moral support to her lover of many years, King Charles VII of France, in his ongoing campaign against English invaders. But this journey had an added impetus. Though the details are unclear, Agnes urgently wanted to warn the king of a plot against him. Whatever she told him, however, her royal lover didn't take it seriously.

Shortly afterward, she went into premature labor and gave birth to her fourth child with the king. While her other three pregnancies had produced full-term, healthy offspring, this child died soon after. Now, on February 9, 1450, Agnes was tortured by a "flux of the belly"—nonstop diarrhea. After two or three days of agony, she whispered of her ravaged body, "It is a little thing and soiled, and smelling of our frailty," and closed her eyes forever.

Rumors flew immediately that the Lady of Beauty, as Agnes was known, had been poisoned. If she had died of a "bloody flux"—hemorrhaging of the uterus, which killed many women after childbirth—suspicions of foul play would have been dampened somewhat. But fatal dysentery in childbirth was strange.

Everyone knew the king's temperamental son and heir, the future Louis XI, despised his father's mistress, blaming her for his falling-out with the king and all the ills of the nation. The prince had been in open revolt against his father for four years. But had he, from his exile hundreds of miles away, found a way to poison her? Perhaps. A 2005 exhumation of Agnes's mortal remains has revealed off-the-charts levels of mercury poisoning—between ten thousand and a hundred thousand times higher than normal.

Born into the lesser nobility, as a teen Agnes served as lady-in-waiting to Isabelle of Lorraine at her court in northeastern France. During a visit, King Charles, who had been deeply depressed, was, according to contemporary reports, struck dumb at the sight of Agnes's stunning beauty. She had golden hair, large, wide blue eyes, and a luscious figure. It was love at first sight—at least, on his part.

King Charles was not a man to inspire the tender fancies of lovely girls, and indeed, his only attractive feature was his crown. Small and slight, he wore heavily padded tunics to hide his sunken chest and narrow shoulders, and in an age where crotch-high tunics were the height of fashion, he wisely wore long robes to conceal his knock-knees. His portrait by Jean Fouquet portrays him as a sad circus clown whose pin head rises above a flood of grotesquely padded red velvet. Considering that royal portraits are almost universally flattering, we can only imagine what the poor man really looked like.

Nor did he offer charisma, charm, or intellect, those qualities that can render appealing the plainest face and most ungainly figure. His father, King Charles VI, had been a madman who stabbed his friends in fits of paranoid rage, and his mother, Isabeau of Bavaria, was an adulteress who sold out France—and her son—to the English. Sometimes Charles sank under the weight of his heredity, mutating into a morbid sloth unwilling to lift a finger against English invaders. At times his nerves were so frayed he couldn't bear anyone to look at him. Mistrustful and terrified, he lived in constant fear of assassination.

It was the women in his life who roused him from his paralyzing torpor, earning him the nickname "Charles the Well-Served." Joan of Arc turned the tide of the Hundred Years' War for him, vanquishing the English. His mother-in-law, Yolande of Aragon, who had raised him since the age of ten, gave him wise counsel. And shrewd Yolande, recognizing the king's obvious infatuation for Agnes, brought the girl into the royal court to be his mistress, even though he was married to Yolande's daughter, Marie of Anjou.

Agnes—probably coached by Yolande—shook Charles from his bouts of debilitating apathy, giving him strength, decisiveness, and confidence. She persuaded him to appoint sage advisers to deal with the war and the pitiful state of the pillaged French economy. Part of Agnes's efforts involved promoting French fashion, selling not only the concept of France as a cultured nation, but also marketing its stylish luxury products abroad. Her gowns were daringly low cut, her perfumed trains up to twenty-five feet long. Her clothing was edged with fur, usually ermine, and her hennins—the tall pointy caps of fairy tales—were several feet high. She glittered with diamonds and emeralds.

Portraits show Agnes following the fashion of plucking the hair around her face to create a larger forehead, and plucking her eyebrows almost entirely off. The earliest surviving portrait of a royal mistress is of Agnes, painted in 1449, a time when secular portraits were not yet common, and many of the rich and famous still bribed church artists to paint their heads on saints. Oddly enough, Agnes was painted as the Virgin Mary, one admirably firm, dazzlingly white breast exposed. Naturally, the pious at court fulminated over the excesses of this fallen woman, as did some nobles. One contemporary wrote, "She displayed in her costumes everything that could lead to ribaldry and dissolute thoughts. She was always desirous of this and stopped at nothing, for she uncovered her shoulders and bosom as far down as the middle of the breast."

Though Agnes clearly reveled in the luxuries of her position, she was known for her kindness. Her five extant letters deal with helping the unfortunate as well as injured animals. Her contemporary, Monstrelet the Chronicler, wrote of her, "So this Agnes was of a very charitable way of life and liberal in alms-giving, and of her possessions she distributed widely to the poor, to the churches and to beggars."

But the king's son, Louis, cared nothing for her kindness and hated her with all the force of his tempestuous soul. His mother, Queen Marie, didn't seem to mind Agnes's hold over the king. Ferret-faced, pious, and the mother of fourteen children, she even stood as godmother to Agnes's three royal bastards, while Louis bristled with rage at the dishonor. Highly intelligent and a born warrior, at seventeen he took charge of the defense of the Languedoc region in southern France against the English. Impatient to succeed his father, whom he saw as weak and wasteful, he criticized Charles's policy and excoriated the royal mistress who had far more influence over the king than he did.

Louis blamed Agnes for his estrangement with his father. One day in 1444, the prince ran into Agnes in the palace, cried, "By our Lord's passion, this woman is the cause of all our misfortunes," and punched her in the face.

When the king banished Louis from his presence, the dauphin tried to lead a rebellion that was quickly put down. Charles exiled his son to southeastern France, where he ruled as a sovereign, and ruled well. But he never stopped plotting against his father and set servants to spy on Agnes. When the king sent men to arrest him, Louis jumped out a window and made his way to the court of Burgundy. There he wrote Charles that he would return, but only on the condition that Charles exile Agnes, not a request likely to find favor with the sovereign.

The dauphin said to his companions, "The king manages his affairs as badly as possible. I intend to put things in order. When I return, I shall drive away Agnes and shall put an end to all his follies and things will go much better than they are now." Perhaps it was a new plot of the dauphin's that Agnes warned King Charles about. And maybe that is why Louis, who had numerous servants of Agnes's in his pay—and possibly her physician—struck when he did.

MODERN POSTMORTEM AND DIAGNOSIS

In 2005, a team of twenty-two researchers from eighteen laboratories exhumed the remains of the lovely royal mistress in the church of Saint-Ours, in Loches. Agnes had been first exhumed back in 1777, when the canons of the church decided it was scandalous for a fallen woman to rest in the choir of their church. Though her wooden coffin had rotted and her lead coffin disintegrated, they found her skull in decent condition, with golden hair drawn into a heavy braid in the back with a long lock on either side. She had plenty of teeth, which those present shamelessly yanked from the jaws and pocketed as souvenirs. The bones were swept into a sandstone urn, which was placed under her black marble effigy in the nave of the church. Her remains were rifled once more during the French Revolution when, most likely, any items of jewelry were plundered, as well as several more teeth. The black marble funerary slab over her heart—which had been buried separately from her body—was taken by a butcher who proceeded to use it as a meat-cutting table in his shop.

The research team found her cranial vault in fair condition with pre-served sections of the face, temples, sinuses, and upper jaw. The back of the skull was missing, probably slipped into someone's pocket. X-rays showed Agnes had a deviated septum and most likely snored. All the teeth in the upper and lower jaw still in place at death had been removed, though seven teeth were mixed in with other remains lower in the urn. They showed little signs of wear, a young age at death, no cavities, low tartar, and a good state of enamel. The team found a jumble of long bones along with bits of mummified muscles, chunks of mummified flesh with hair and eyebrows still attached, and, as the French scientists so poetically put it, "putrefaction juice." A strange, sweet odor rose from the remains, spooking the researchers.

To authenticate the identity of the remains, the team carbon-dated them to the year of her death exactly, 1450. Then, using a computer, a paleopathologist superimposed the skull fragments on the face of Agnes's effigy, which had been sculpted from life. The researchers found a perfect alignment of the bones with the sculpture: the shape of the chin, the placement of the teeth, the position of her ear canals, the opening of the nostrils, the size of the nasal cavity, and the distance and shape of her eyes all matched. What they didn't find was the plucking of eyebrows and hairline to the extent shown in her portraits. Artists had exaggerated that fashion.

Additional tests confirmed that Agnes had extremely white skin and ate a mixed diet of meat and vegetables. Her hair had been stained black by lead from the deteriorating coffin but cleaned up as blond. And there was no evidence of malaria or any other disease. But scientists did find numerous intestinal roundworm eggs, common enough in that time. Roundworms are intestinal parasites that grow up to ten inches long and live in colonies throughout the digestive tract. Agnes must have suffered from abdominal pain, bloody stool, weight loss, and diarrhea.

In the urn, researchers also found remains of a male fern, a plant often combined with small amounts of quicksilver to combat roundworms in the Middle Ages. Clearly, Agnes was receiving treatment for her condition.

But when scientists studied Agnes's hair—from her head, her armpits, and her pubic region—they found mind-boggling concentrations of mercury: ten thousand to one hundred thousand times the normal amount, many thousands of times more than she would have ingested as worm medication. Nor had the mercury been slathered on Agnes as part of the embalming process. The poison was inside her perfectly preserved root sheaths, with no mercury at all on the outside. Researchers determined that Agnes ingested the mercury between forty-eight and seventy-two hours before her death, right around the time she first became ill. Mercury poisoning was most certainly what killed her.

Scientists examining the mush in the bottom of the urn discovered that during embalming, Agnes's abdominal cavity had been filled with grains, berries, aromatic spices, black pepper, fragrant leaves, and mulberry twigs. This was the source of the strange aroma sweetening the air as soon as they opened the urn. They also found the tiny bones of an infant of seven months' gestation. They could not determine if mercury poisoning caused the premature birth of the baby, or if Agnes was poisoned during or after labor. What must be certain is that Agnes's doctor, Robert Poitevin, personal physician to the king and the top medical professional in all France, would never have accidentally given her such a massive and fatal dose of mercury. And physicians, as we know from Cangrande della Scala, are in a unique position to intentionally poison their victims. Their patients trusted them. Kings and queens refrained from using tasters and meekly drank whatever concoctions their physicians handed them or freely offered up their royal rear ends for what they assumed would be a salubrious enema.

Naturally, Agnes's death sparked rumors of poisoning. As the contemporary chronicler Jacques Leclerc wrote in his memoirs, "And they said too that the said dauphin had caused the death of a lady named Agnes who was the fairest woman in the kingdom and greatly in love with the king, his father." But Charles could hardly charge his dashing, popular son and heir with her murder.

Without Agnes by his side, the king slipped back into slothful melancholy, rousing himself long enough to arrange brilliant marriages to French aristocrats for his three daughters with Agnes. For a decade after her death, he engaged in wine-soaked orgies in between debilitating bouts of illness. Finally, an infection in his jaw—perhaps from a rotten tooth—caused an abscess to develop in his mouth. The growth swelled to such proportions that the king could no longer eat or drink. Charles VII starved to death in 1461.

9

EDWARD VI, KING of ENGLAND, 1537–1553

The fifteen-year-old king lay in bed, his head and feet grotesquely swollen. Scabs and sores covered his body, and his hair had fallen out in clumps. His fingernails and toenails had turned black and come off. He couldn't sleep, could barely breathe, and vomited everything he ate. Burning up with fever and racked by violent coughing, he spat up matter that "is sometimes colored a greenish yellow and black, sometimes pink, like the color of blood," according to one witness. Another reported, "The sputum which he brings up is livid, black, fetid and full of carbon; it smells beyond measure; if it is put in a basin full of water it sinks to the bottom . . . To the doctors all these things portend death." His symptoms were sure signs of poison, many believed.

The wretched, sweat-soaked creature coughing on the bed was the vaunted heir of Henry VIII, the future of the Tudor dynasty that the king had spent nearly thirty years trying to conceive. Having divorced his first wife for not giving him a son and beheaded his second for the same reason, Henry took as his third wife an English noblewoman named Jane Seymour. Sixteen months after the wedding, Jane accomplished what her predecessors could not: she produced the long-desired heir, Edward.

All the church bells in London pealed out their exuberant joy at his birth on October 12, 1537. A male heir meant national stability, safety from the civil wars that had devastated England in the previous century. But the exultation was tempered by the death of Queen Jane on October 23, probably from puerperal fever caused by her doctors' dirty hands and crusty instruments.

The prince grew to be a handsome boy with pale blond hair and blue-gray eyes. Chancellor Thomas Audley had never seen "so goodly a child of his age, so merry, so pleasant, so good and loving countenance." When the prince was four, the French ambassador described him as "handsome, well-fed and remarkably tall for his age."

Edward was raised in the lap of Tudor luxury. His knives and spoons were studded with precious gems; his napkins sported gold and silver lace. The finest Flemish tapestries hung from his walls. Even the covers of his books were of gold, sparkling with rubies and diamonds. A French visitor recorded that when the little boy, shining in cloth of gold and silver and adorned with diamonds, pearls, and emeralds, walked about, he lit up entire rooms as the light struck him. His dagger, glowing with gemstones, hung from his belt by a rope of fat pearls. But Edward was no obnoxious spoiled princeling. He was a serious scholar, endeavoring to please his tutors and, most of all, his father. From an early age, he showed great interest in the religious questions convulsing England.

When Edward was nine, Henry ate one too many pork chops and died. He had made a will to create a regency council consisting of sixteen members with equal authority. But these gentlemen were lavishly bribed by Edward's uncle, Edward Seymour, to cede him complete power as Lord Protector of the Realm and Governor of the King's Person. Thus the real ruler of England was not the "godly imp," as many called the adorable nine-year-old king, but his uncle, who immediately rewarded himself with the august title and accompanying wealth of Duke of Somerset. His arrogance and incompetence, however, soon alienated many. The ambassador of the Holy Roman Empire, François van der Delft, wrote that Somerset was "looked down upon by everybody as a dry, sour, opinionated man."

The duke's administration soon sank into chaos due to deteriorating economic conditions and increasing religious contention. He even beheaded his own brother, Thomas, for attempting to kidnap the king and wield power himself. Somerset's bitter enemy on the council, John Dudley, Earl of Warwick, staged a coup on October 7, 1549, and had Somerset executed in January 1552. He purged his rival's supporters and generously rewarded his own, loading them with titles and lands even as he made himself Duke of Northumberland.

Throughout these years of adults behaving badly, Edward remained a well-behaved, studious young man, devoted to becoming the best king he could be. One courtier described him as "the beautifullest creature that liveth under the sun, the wittiest, the most amiable and the gentlest thing of all the world. Such a spirit of capacity, learning the thing taught him by his schoolmasters, that it is a wonder to hear say."

At the age of twelve, Edward was fluent in Latin, had a good knowledge of Greek, and spoke some Italian and French. His studies included Cicero and Aristotle in their original languages, "but no study delights him more than that of the Holy Scriptures, of which he daily reads about ten chapters with the greatest attention," wrote one reformer. Guided by his council, Edward zealously intended to remove all taint of Catholicism left in the Church of England. Edward's church was sober, biblically focused, and the foundation of what came to be known as Puritanism.

Like his father as a young man, Edward excelled in physical exercise. He jousted, fenced, rode in full armor, hunted tirelessly, and practiced archery. He made frequent use of the tennis courts at Whitehall, Hampton Court, and Greenwich Palace. Records for 1551 indicated he played tennis 293 times.

On April 2, 1552, Edward "fell sick of the measles and the smallpox." He made a swift recovery and on April 12 wrote in his diary, "We have been a little troubled with the small pox . . . but now we have shaken that quite away." Foreign ambassadors noted how quickly he recovered, bursting with health by April 28 and returning to physical exercise in May. The imperial ambassador reported that Edward "takes riding exercise and fences daily, without forgoing his studies, which are multiple, and concern especially the new religion, in which he is said to be proficient. He has begun to be present at the Council and to attend to certain affairs himself."

In October 1552, Edward developed a cough and grew weak. The illness did not seem serious, however, and by Christmas the court heaved a collective sigh of relief to see him recovered. But in February 1553, the imperial ambassador reported that Edward was ill again: "He suffers a good deal when the fever is upon him, especially from a difficulty in drawing his breath, which is due to the compression of the organs on the right side."

For weeks, Edward stayed in his room as grave-faced physicians came and went. Despite two brief periods of seeming recovery, by the middle of May, he was seriously ill again. He spat up a rainbow of sputum—green, black, yellow, and dark pink. His doctors believed he suffered from a "suppurating tumor" on the lungs, which caused the racking cough and high fever. The imperial ambassador wrote that the king was still "indisposed, and it is held for certain that he cannot escape."

Oozing ulcers spread across Edward's body. Some stayed open, while others hardened into scabs. Mottled purple bruises appeared all over his body, as if someone had beaten him badly. He was wasting away, yet his head and feet were grotesquely swollen. The imperial ambassador wrote, "He does not sleep except when he be stuffed with drugs, which doctors call opiates . . . first one thing then another are given him, but the doctors do not exceed twelve grains at a time, for these drugs are never given by doctors unless the patient is in great pain, or tormented by constant sleeplessness, or racked by violent coughing."

Edward must have realized his illness could be fatal and, perhaps at the instigation of Northumberland, devised his own plan for succession to the throne. As the king told his shocked council gathered around his sickbed, he did not wish to comply with Henry VIII's will in giving the crown to his oldest sister, Princess Mary, if he died without legitimate children, and to his next sister, Princess Elizabeth, if Mary died childless. Edward wanted to disinherit them both with a stroke of the pen.

Catholic Mary, Edward knew, "would provoke great disturbances," and "it would be all over for the religion whose fair foundation we have laid." He had often argued with Mary about her stubborn insistence on hearing Mass. Nor did he wish Elizabeth to inherit because, even though brother and sister were close and she was Protestant, she was "a bastard and sprung from an illegitimate bed." Edward declared that both sisters would be given 1,000 pounds annually "to live in quiet order" and would receive a one-time payment of 10,000 pounds if they married according to the council's wishes.

Who, then, would inherit the crown? It would descend through the heirs of Frances, Duchess of Suffolk, daughter of Henry VIII's younger sister Mary. Frances had no sons, but the eldest of her three daughters, Jane Grey, already a zealous religious reformer at sixteen, would be the next queen of England. On May 25, Northumberland married his son Guildford to Jane, making him the future king.

For months, rumors had abounded that someone was slowly poisoning the king, hoping to make his death look like a long, drawn-out illness. Reformers blamed the Catholics who wanted Mary on the throne, knowing she would bring back the pope, monasteries, and saints' relics in a heartbeat. But the imperial ambassador heard that many people blamed Northumberland, a "great Tyrant," for poisoning Edward. The young king, poised to take power into his own hands, had given clear evidence of a strong personality and would do things his own way. Northumberland stood to lose power as Edward grew older. But with his son as King Guildford, he would retain it.

On June 25, Edward was so ill that it seemed certain he would die. The imperial ambassador wrote, "It is firmly believed that he will die tomorrow, for he has not the strength to stir, and can hardly breathe. His body no longer performs its functions, his nails and hair are dropping off, and all his person is scabby."

Yet he held on into the new month. Between eight and nine o'clock on the night of July 6, 1553, Edward's breathing grew labored and ragged. He raised his eyes upward and gasped, "O Lord God save thy chosen people of England! O my Lord God, defend this realm from papistry, and maintain thy true religion, that I and my people may praise thy holy name, for thy Son Jesus Christ's sake!" One of his gentlemen took the boy in his arms. "I am faint," the king said. "Lord have mercy upon me and take my spirit." And He did.

Henry Machyn, a London clothier, wrote in his diary entry for July 6 that "the noble king Edward the VI . . . was poisoned as everybody says." The French ambassador reported that those who whispered that the king had been poisoned had been placed in the Tower. An Italian observer noted that there had been "suspicions here and there thrown out that he was gradually carried off by some slow poison administered long before."

CONTEMPORARY POSTMORTEM

Rumor notwithstanding, during Edward's autopsy, surgeons found that "the disease whereof his majesty died was the disease of the lungs." They found large cavities in the lungs "which had in them two great ulcers and were putrefied, by means whereof he fell into consumption, and so hath he wasted, being utterly incurable."

THE UNLIKELIHOOD OF A MODERN POSTMORTEM

Edward's remains are sealed in the vaults beneath Westminster Abbey, unlikely ever to be studied. Queen Elizabeth II, bolstered in her stance by the Church of England, steadfastly refuses to disinter her ancestors. Responding to a request to open some tombs in Westminster Abbey for research, in 1995 the Very Reverend Michael Mayne, Dean of Westminster, said huffily, "I do not believe we are in the business of satisfying curiosity."

Because the British monarchy is based on the royal bloodline, it faces a dilemma when it comes to studying royal remains. What if DNA proves that a dead king was not related to his father? Would that mean Elizabeth II was not the legitimate queen?

A modern analysis of the bones of two children found under a staircase in the Tower in 1674 could prove if they are the remains of the lost princes, twelve-year-old King Edward V and his brother, nine-year-old Richard, Duke of York. In 1483, the boys vanished in the Tower while in the care of their uncle, who immediately proclaimed himself King Richard III and never publicly mentioned them again. Charles II had the bones interred together in an urn and placed near the remains of the little princes' relatives below the Henry VII Lady Chapel in Westminster Abbey. Repeated requests from researchers to study the bones have been denied.

The 2012 discovery of the remains of King Richard III in a parking lot was a godsend to scientists, who could examine them to their heart's content. If they had been found on royal property, it is likely they never would have been studied. Doctors determined that the skeleton belonged to a man about Richard's age at death—thirty-three—with severe scoliosis of the spine—which also fits historical reports—and numerous skull injuries, which was how Richard reportedly died.

Most shockingly, what the royal family feared all along did, in fact, come to pass. Tests conducted to match the skeleton's DNA to that of descendants of Richard's sister, Anne of York, confirmed a direct line of mitochondrial DNA passed from mother to daughter. As for the male side of the family, Richard's DNA should have matched that of cousins going back to a common ancestor. John of Gaunt, who died in 1399, was the father of King Henry IV and Richard's great-grandfather— at least in the history books. But when researchers studied the DNA of living members of the ducal Beaufort family—also supposedly descended from John of Gaunt—they found a break, euphemistically called a "false paternity event." While Beaufort family members point to a raucous eighteenth-century duchess, some scholars believe that Henry IV was a bastard passed off on John of Gaunt, which would mean that all English kings since 1399 had no genetic right to rule.

Researchers could determine exactly when the false paternity event occurred if given access to the tombs of those individuals descending from John of Gaunt to the living Beauforts, but such an investigation is not likely to recommend itself to Her Majesty Queen Elizabeth II. Most people assume the reason for such refusals is that the British royal family nobly wishes the dead to rest in peace.

Before the advent of DNA testing, however, British researchers gleefully cracked open coffins and handled the remains. In 1789, workers restoring St. George's Chapel at Windsor Castle found the coffin of Edward IV, the father of the lost princes, who died in 1483. The skeletal remains included long brown hair and reddish-brown liquid in the bottom of the coffin. Members of the public visiting the tomb plucked out bones, snipped off hair, and scooped up the liquid as souvenirs. In 1813, a group of gentlemen including George, Prince of Wales, opened up the vault of Charles I, who had been beheaded in 1649, cracked open his coffin, and held up his head for inspection. They noted that he looked just like his portraits by Anthony van Dyke, except his nose was missing.

In 1868, at the pinnacle of Victorian prudery and decorum, researchers investigated the chaotic vaults beneath Westminster Abbey to determine exactly who was there and, if possible, get a good look at dead kings and queens. James I had rammed himself into Henry VII's vault, thrusting aside Henry's wife, Elizabeth of York, as if to emphasize his descent from the first Tudor king. Elizabeth I's coffin was plunked on top of her half sister, Mary I, as if to proclaim herself the victor in death as she had been in life.

Nearby, in a lonely little vault only seven feet long and two feet wide, the investigators discovered Edward. It was one of the leakiest spots in the underground tombs, and his coffin was "rent and deformed as well as wasted by long corrosion," according to the report. It was so corroded, in fact, that the investigators could see his smooth, pale skull.

MODERN DIAGNOSIS

Even without scientific analysis, we can deduce what killed the teenage king. Tuberculosis was rampant in Tudor England. It had killed Edward's grandfather, Henry VII, at fifty-two, and it may have been what killed Edward's uncle, Arthur, Prince of Wales, also at fifteen. If Edward inhaled the mycobacterium tuberculosis into his lungs years earlier, when he was perfectly healthy, his immune system would have fought off the infection by walling it off or encapsulating it. Called latent tuberculosis, the bacteria would have been alive but dormant, unable to spread to surrounding tissues in the lungs or into the bloodstream. And neither Edward nor his doctors would have known of his exposure.

If the immune system of a person with latent tuberculosis becomes suppressed, the walled-off bacteria can reactivate, obliterating the wall. Edward's agonizing decline could have been caused by his contracting measles in April 1552. Though he bounced back quickly to ride and joust and hunt, measles—now known to reduce the body's natural resistance to tuberculosis—could have launched the bacteria racing through his body. By February of the following year, it had damaged his lungs enough to keep him in bed with coughing fits.

Edward's body would have resisted this onslaught by releasing chemicals into the blood to fight the infection, triggering fever and inflammation. As the weeks passed, the raging infection became sepsis, damaging his organs and causing open sores to form on his skin and his hair and nails to fall out. As his lungs became ever more damaged, they no longer functioned properly, causing cyanosis, a deficiency of oxygen in the blood that discolors the skin, creating the appearance of bruises. Active tuberculosis causes abscesses filled with pus to form in the lungs, which was what the physicians found during the autopsy.

While the royal doctors recognized consumption when they saw it, both in living and in autopsied patients, they had no idea what caused it. The tubercle bacillus wasn't identified until 1882 by the German doctor Robert Koch. It's safe to agree that Edward was indeed poisoned, not by arsenic but by a massive infection. The royal doctors—though they would not have understood the progress of the illness—came close to naming the correct cause of death.

Soon after Edward's death, Northumberland massed troops to make sure Jane Grey and his son took the throne. The long-suffering Princess Mary, who had great popular support, raised her own troops and, after nine days, routed Northumberland and reclaimed her birthright. The duke, his son, and Jane Grey lost their heads.

Most historians focus on the enthralling reigns of Edward's relatives: Henry VII's roll of dynastic dice in the bloody battle of Bosworth Field. Henry VIII mooning the pope and killing his wives. Bloody Mary's bonfire of the heretics. The Virgin Queen soundly defeating the Spanish Armada. Alas, history treats Edward as a Tudor footnote. We can only imagine what his reign would have been like had he lived into his prime. Given his sense of justice and responsibility, his scholarship and ardor for hard work, he may have been one of the best kings ever. One public eulogy lamented, "For age he might deserve a riper end. Death calls the best, and leaves the worse to mend."

10

JEANNE d'ALBRET, QUEEN of NAVARRE, 1528–1572

On June 4, 1572, Jeanne d'Albret, the forty-three-year-old queen of Navarre, was reputedly poisoned, not at a banquet, the usual place for secret assassination, but during a Paris shopping expedition. Her death would, by the end of the summer, play a part in unleashing waves of violence that would forever stain the reputation of the French royal family.

Queen Jeanne, the leader of the Huguenot movement in France, spent the day visiting the trendiest boutiques with her political and religious enemy, Catherine de Medici, the powerful Catholic queen mother of France. An important wedding was coming up, and for the several days of festivities the two queens would need new gowns, jewels, ruffs, gloves, perfumes, and cosmetics.

Jeanne must have found shopping with Catherine quite a chore. Not only did Jeanne eschew the sinful vanities of fashion, wearing the simple black and white gowns of a pious Huguenot widow, but the upcoming wedding broke her heart. The groom was her only son, eighteen-year-old Henri, likeable, witty, and brave, who had successfully commanded an army at fifteen. Though he clearly had an eye for the ladies, Jeanne had raised him as a good Puritan—prayer, sermons, no gambling, dancing, or anything approaching fun.

The bride was Princess Marguerite, Catherine's stunning nineteen-year-old daughter, extravagant in dress, brazenly flirtatious, and devoutly Catholic, to Jeanne's mind a Jezebel, the Red Whore of Babylon. "As for her picture, I'll send you one from Paris," she had promised her son a few months earlier.

> She is beautiful, discreet and graceful, but she has grown up in the most vicious and corrupt atmosphere imaginable. I cannot see that anyone escapes its poison . . . Not for anything on earth would I have you come to live here. Therefore, I wish you to be married and to retire—with your wife—from this corruption. Although I knew it was bad, I find it even worse than I feared. Here women make advances to men rather than the other way around . . . The men cover themselves with jewels. The king just spent 100,000 écus on gems and buys more every day.

To a friend, Jeanne wrote, "As for the beauty of Madame [Marguerite], I admit she has a good figure, but it is too tightly corseted. Her face is spoiled by too much makeup, which displeases me."

Marguerite was as appalled by the wedding as Jeanne. She saw Henri as a bandy-legged, wisecracking smart-ass who smelled like a goat and who had a nose larger than his kingdom. Marguerite liked dashing, haughty cavaliers, and throughout a long life of spirited nymphomania, she would have sex with almost all of them. Her union with Henri would be a political marriage of opposites in every sense of the word, roping numerous people who hated one another into one big, miserable family.

Catherine insisted on the marriage because she believed it would end the civil religious war bleeding France dry. And there was a more personal reason. Her astrologer, Nostradamus, had predicted that none of her sons would have legitimate male offspring. Their distant cousin, Jeanne's son, Henri, would become king of France, and *his* descendants would rule for generations. Catherine believed that if her daughter were Henri's wife, then those of her blood would still sit on the throne. Jeanne had refused to sanction the match—or mismatch—for several years. Finally, wily Catherine tightened the noose around Jeanne's neck, threatening to have the pope declare Henri illegitimate because of

Jeanne's first, annulled marriage to a German prince. Jeanne was forced to relent, sending her son to Sodom.

Jeanne was the only child of Henri d'Albret, king of Navarre, and Marguerite d'Angouleme, sister of King François I. Navarre was a blip of a kingdom only fifty miles by thirty-seven squeezed in between France and Spain. Intelligent and studious as a child, Jeanne grew into an attractive young woman with light brown hair and pale blue eyes. Her nose was long and slender, her face lit by a vivacious intelligence. She had a sprightly figure, which she would keep until her death. After the marriage she had made at the age of twelve was annulled, at nineteen she wed the dashing, thirty-year-old Antoine de Bourbon, duc de Vendôme, a cousin of the new king, Henri II.

Antoine was a renowned warrior who swaggered into Jeanne's life smelling of enemy blood and cannon smoke, a heady perfume that most women found irresistible. A contemporary wrote that Jeanne had "no pleasure or occupation except in talking about or writing to [her husband]. She does it in company and in private . . . the waters cannot quench the flame of her love."

But Antoine was a spendthrift womanizer, and not terribly bright, which quickly quenched the flame of Jeanne's love. When her father died in 1555, she became the ruling queen of Navarre, but Antoine, as king, meddled and made deals behind her back, even offering to give her kingdom to Spain in return for a better kingdom for himself—Milan, perhaps. Antoine not only disgusted his wife, he became a laughingstock to his peers. One contemporary said that he had "nothing but real women and imaginary crowns in his head."

Jeanne found solace in a new religion spreading across France. The Geneva-based Frenchman Jehan Cauvin—known to history as John Calvin—sent ministers throughout Europe preaching a no-nonsense message: Christians can have a direct relationship with God without priests or saints to intercede for them. They should read the Bible in their native tongue. The statues and paintings in Catholic churches go directly against the biblical command not to worship images.

Jeanne, now the mother of Henri, born in 1553, and Catherine, born in 1559, officially converted in 1560 and devoted herself to Calvinism with her ferocious logic and "frightening brain," as the Venetian ambassador termed it. She championed freedom of worship for Huguenots, outlawed Catholic services in her domains, and encouraged people to destroy the images in churches, whitewash the walls, and read the Bible in French. Calvinist services were celebrated not only throughout Navarre but across France—and usually tolerated by Catherine, whose political outlook was all about pragmatic balance.

But civil war broke out as Huguenots insisted on more rights while Catholics wanted them to have none at all. Antoine, who had changed religions several times for his financial advantage, died fighting for the Catholics, probably to Jeanne's relief. By 1569, the royal Catholic army was bankrupt and riddled with famine, fever, and extraordinarily stupid generals. France was cannibalizing itself, grower weaker every day. Catherine, realizing Mars wasn't helping her, decided perhaps Venus could and started her charm offensive on Jeanne to persuade her to agree to the marriage.

Finally, in the spring of 1572, Jeanne capitulated and went to Paris to discuss the wedding. She and Catherine argued about every detail: where it would be held, who would be invited, who would officiate, and what rites and rituals would be used.

Jeanne, exhausted by the unending arguments, wrote Henri, "I do not know how I can stand it, they scratch me, they stick pins into me, they flatter me, they tear out my fingernails, without letup. I am badly lodged, holes have been drilled into the walls of my apartment, and Madame d'Uzes [one of Catherine's ladies] spies on me." She added, with an ominous note, "I fear that I may fall sick, for I do not feel at all well."

Finally, everything was decided. On March 25, Jeanne wrote her son, "Every enticement will be offered to debauch you, in everything from your appearance to your religion . . . Set up an invincible resistance against this. I know it is their object because they do not conceal it." She added some motherly advice: "Try to train your hair to stand up and be sure there are no lice in it."

Dispirited and fatigued, by late May Jeanne began the wedding shopping. She wasn't just buying clothing for herself. Henri, whom she had kept as much as possible in the country, needed courtly clothing. For years, courtiers had laughed at his provincial ways and country twang. She was also expected to buy clothing and jewelry for her future daughter-in-law, that tart, Marguerite.

On that Wednesday, June 4, Jeanne decided to splurge and buy herself a little something she would truly enjoy. Though the thin-lipped puritanical matron was not given to self-indulgence, she had always loved perfumed gloves. In an age when the most glittering courtiers stank of body odor, people perfumed just about anything they could. Gloves, in particular, required plenty of fragrance. To turn stiff, hairy hide into supple, buttery leather, tanners used copious amounts of animal excrement, which left in its wake a pungent, rancid reek. Gloves were scented with cloves, musk, ambergris, orange blossom, violets, jasmine, and even kitchen herbs such as thyme and rosemary.

Queen Catherine took Jeanne to buy gloves at a trendy boutique in the heart of the Paris shopping district owned by her personal perfumer. Master René Bianco was a Florentine who had traveled with Catherine forty years earlier on her journey to wed Prince Henri. A Medici retainer who cooked up recipes in his basement laboratory, however, was doomed to have the reputation of a poisoner. Rumor had it that Queen Catherine, who was never well liked as a foreigner and banker's daughter, used Master René's more nefarious concoctions to poison her enemies. And, indeed, many people died at the French court.

Shrugging aside such rumors, Jeanne bought a pair of gloves from the perfumer. Perhaps she wore them out of the store. She certainly must have tried them on for fit and sniffed their lilting, exuberant scent. By the time she returned home, she felt unwell and went to bed with a slight fever. After a restless night, she woke with a higher fever and a terrible pain in the upper right side of her chest. The physicians were called but could offer her no relief. By June 6, she had difficulty breathing.

The king sent his own physicians, but they, too, were powerless to help Jeanne. Weakening by the hour, she drew up a new will. As her friends cried around her bed, she told them not to weep, for God was calling her to a better life.

A Huguenot minister said, "See Madame, with the eye of faith, Jesus Christ the Savior, seated on His Father's right hand, is holding out his arms to receive you. Do you not wish to go to him?"

Jeanne said, "Yes, much more willingly, I assure you, than to remain in this world where I see nothing but vanity." Despite her agony, she remained calm and lucid until her last hour.

The morning of Monday, June 9, she lay quietly with her eyes closed, apparently without suffering. Suddenly a spasm of pain gripped her. Two of her ladies raised her in their arms as she gasped for breath. Her hands and feet became ice cold. Her alarmed physician instructed them to rub her chest to keep her warm. She had lost the power of speech and slipped away between eight and nine o'clock, aged forty-three.

The sudden death of the leader of the Huguenot cause came as a great blow to religious reformers. The Venetian ambassador wrote, "She was a very bold woman and her death is causing the greatest possible setback to Huguenot affairs." However, the papal nuncio, Fabio Mirto Frangipani, crowed with glee when he wrote the pope on the day of Jeanne's death, "In a great proof of God's almighty power, on this day of Corpus Christi, the Queen of Navarre died in this city, this morning, on the fifth day of her illness . . . at a time when the Huguenots were most happy to have their Queen here and she was most triumphant, preparing for her son's wedding . . . and other evils for God's dishonor and the disturbance of Christian states. But God—may He be forever praised!—snatched suddenly . . . such an important enemy of His most Holy Church."

Many in France and across Europe believed the sinister Catherine had arranged with Master René to sell Jeanne poison-drenched gloves. But Catherine, though she disliked the prickly, prudish Jeanne, had finally gotten her way with the marriage. And there were others who hated Jeanne with a vitriolic fury—the pope, for instance, and His Most Catholic Majesty, King Philip II of Spain.

CONTEMPORARY POSTMORTEM

A Paris surgeon named Desnoeds performed the autopsy the night of June 9 in the presence of Jeanne's personal physician, who was also a Huguenot, and several other physicians, "at the command of the Queen." He found all of Jeanne's organs in perfect condition except her lungs, which had hardened and showed extensive damage. On her upper right lung—the spot where she had suffered excruciating pain in her last days—they found a large abscess that had broken, leaking pus into her lungs.

Laying down his bloody knife, Desnoeds said, "Messieurs, if her majesty had died, as it has been wrongly alleged, from having smelled some poisoned object, the marks would be perceptible on the coating of the brain, but on the contrary, the brain is as healthful and free from injury as possible. If her majesty had died from swallowing poison, traces of such would have been visible in the stomach. We can discover nothing of the kind. There is no other cause, therefore, for her majesty's decease, but the rupture of an abscess on the lungs."

MODERN DIAGNOSIS

It is likely that Jeanne suffered from low-grade, chronic tuberculosis since childhood. Family letters mention her periodic bouts of coughing and spitting up blood, during which she rested in bed for a week or two. Frequently, she visited health spas to take the restorative waters. It seems that finally her infection, perhaps worsened by the stress of the upcoming wedding, rose to a fatal level.

Jeanne had instructed that she be buried next to her father in the cathedral of Lescar, a town in Navarre. She would have been furious to realize that Catherine had her interred next to her despised husband, Antoine, in Vendôme. In 1793, ransacking revolutionaries stripped the bodies of both Jeanne and Antoine of valuables and tossed them into a ditch.

Jeanne's death paved the way for the infamous St. Bartholomew's Day Massacre, which for centuries has been a byword for Catholic infamy. Upon her death, Admiral Gaspard II de Coligny became the leader of the Huguenots and went to Paris with thousands of his followers for the August 18 wedding of Henri and Marguerite. But on August 22, when Coligny was shot and wounded in the street by an unknown assailant, Queen Catherine and her son, twenty-two-year-old King Charles IX, feared the restive Huguenots would rise up against them. Everyone believed Catherine had poisoned Jeanne with the gloves, no matter what the autopsy revealed. And now someone had tried to kill Jeanne's replacement.

The king and his mother ordered the assassination of some thirty Huguenot leaders in Paris. Seeing the violence, many Parisians took it into their own hands to kill their Protestant neighbors. The massacre spread across the city and into the provinces. It is impossible to say how many died, but estimates range from five thousand to seventy thousand. Jeanne's son, Henri, a sword at his throat, expressed his sudden and ardent desire to become Catholic. Hearing of the slaughter, the ultra-Catholic King Philip II of Spain laughed for the only time on record, according to witnesses. But other monarchs were enraged. You know you've gone over the top when Czar Ivan the Terrible of Russia expresses his distaste at your excessive violence.

Henri clowned his way through four years of genteel Catholic imprisonment at court before riding out on a palace hunting expedition and not stopping until he reached Navarre, where he reaffirmed his Protestant faith. His wife eventually joined him, though they despised each other and both openly kept lovers. In 1586, after Marguerite led a rebellion against him, Henri imprisoned her in a fortress for eighteen years. In 1599 he divorced her. In 1589, he became Henri IV of France, fulfilling Jeanne's dreams and Nostradamus's prediction. But with Spanish armies fighting a heretic king and the gates of Paris locked against him, in 1593 Henri decided to convert once again. His mother would have turned over in her grave.

Once, when Henri met an old Huguenot friend coming out of Mass, he asked the man what he was doing there. "I am here because you are, Sire," the man replied. "Oh, I understand," the king retorted, "you have some crown to gain."

11

ERIK XIV, KING of SWEDEN,
1533–1577

On February 22, 1577, the forty-four-year-old deposed King Erik XIV of Sweden dug into a bowl of his favorite pea soup in his genteel prison at Örbyhus Castle, some seventy miles from Stockholm, where his younger half brother, Johan III, had reigned in his stead for nine years. It is not known if the mad former monarch noticed a metallic taste to his soup. But within a few hours, Erik complained of pain in his stomach and chest and took to his bed. At two o'clock on the morning of February 26, he died. Rumor had it his jailer had put arsenic in his pea soup.

It was a pathetic end to a promising life. Erik was the oldest son of King Gustav Vasa, an ambitious young nobleman who had led a rebellion to free Sweden from Danish rule and crowned himself king in 1523. Unlike his rather provincial father, Erik had been born to the purple and received a truly royal education. His Latin was as fluent as his Swedish. He read Hebrew and Greek, and spoke French, Spanish, Italian, Finnish, and German. He was well versed in history and geography and loved tinkering with technological devises. A true Renaissance man, he could draw, play the lute, and compose music.

At the age of twenty-six, Prince Erik decided he wanted to marry the new queen of England, Elizabeth, also twenty-six, and sent her romantic letters. On February 25, 1560, Elizabeth replied politely to his amorous overtures, "While we perceive therefrom that the zeal and love of your mind towards us is not diminished, yet in part we are grieved that we cannot gratify your serene highness with the same kind of affections. We do not conceive in our heart to take a husband." Elizabeth was alarmed that he intended to visit her to woo her in person. She urged him not to because "nothing but expectation can happen to your serene highness in this business." Undeterred, Erik prepared ships full of costly gifts for the journey and rode to the Swedish coast to board one. But then news reached him that his father had died on September 29, 1560. Erik—now Erik XIV—was king. He returned to Stockholm to arrange his father's funeral and his own coronation.

Tall and well built, with reddish-blond hair and a long beard, Erik was a handsome and imposing figure. An able administrator, he took his responsibilities seriously. Indeed, he was too serious, completely lacking his father's humor and earthy bonhomie. He had no friends, as he believed his birth was so superior it would be unfitting to mingle as equals with anyone else, including his younger half brothers and sisters. Worst of all, Erik harbored suspicions that the nobles were planning treachery. Sometimes his mood swung from violent rage to quivering fear.

Despite Elizabeth's continuing, gentle rebuffs, Erik was still obsessed about marrying her. In September 1561, he set sail with an impressive fleet for England where the English people, joyful at the prospect of a royal wedding, sold woodcuts and other souvenirs with both monarchs seated on twin thrones. But for a second time fortune prevented his meeting Elizabeth. After weeks of battling against winds that battered him back to Sweden, he gave up. Indeed, there was much at home for him to attend to. Denmark had never completely accepted the loss of Sweden as a territory, and Erik wanted to end Danish domination of the region. The result was the Northern Seven Years' War, which began in 1563.

In addition to fighting enemies outside his kingdom, Erik waged an internal war on his aristocracy. He insisted on curbing their power, refused to consider their petitions, took away their lands and income, and forced them to pay higher taxes. He saw every little mistake they made—whether by negligence or laziness—as an act of sabotage and treason. His increasingly violent outbursts and punishments created ever-greater anger among the nobles, which in turn made him more paranoid. Erik set up a kangaroo court where commoners served as judges, convicting and fining noblemen for treason, conspiracy, and sedition.

Still smarting from Elizabeth's continuing rejections, the king became enraged when he saw his pages elegantly dressed, fearing all the court ladies would fall in love with them and not him. If anyone put a hand over his mouth to cough, he saw it as whispering rebellion. When Erik's scepter was found broken on the floor of his dressing room, he had his chamberlain arrested for treason. One day, finding a jug, a cloak, and a horse halter on the floor of the royal privy, he condemned two guards to death for trying "to annoy him."

As the years went by, the issue of the king's marriage grew increasingly urgent. In 1567, at thirty-four, with a long line of mistresses and a sprinkling of royal bastards, Erik had no legitimate son. Next in line was his half brother, Johan, who had taken himself out of the running by getting locked up in prison for subversion. The third brother, Magnus, suffered from lunacy even worse than Erik's. At the age of nineteen, he reportedly saw a mermaid in the castle moat, dove off the ramparts, hit the water with a great splash, and nearly drowned. As his servants tried to fish him out, he continued screaming that he wanted to catch the mermaid.

The more Erik thought about it, the more it seemed to him that his enemies had sabotaged his matrimonial chances so he would have no heir and his line would die out. It wasn't just his courtship of Elizabeth that had foundered miserably. He had also been rejected by Mary, Queen of Scots, Anna of Saxony, Christine of Hesse, and Renata of Lorraine. Why should it be so hard for a splendid king like him to get a wife unless everyone was undermining him?

A devotee of astrology, Erik had learned in his horoscope that he would lose his crown to a "light-haired man," which must have driven him crazy considering how many light-haired men there were in Sweden. He began to believe that this light-haired man was Nils Sture, scion of the powerful family who had ruled Sweden as regents for the Danish crown until Erik's father claimed Sweden for himself.

Erik decided that the Stures were behind all the disasters of his reign.

He threw Nils, his father, Svante, and several of their friends and relatives into prison. Then, on May 24, 1567, Erik had a change of heart, fell on his knees before Svante, and begged his forgiveness. Two hours later, the king returned to the castle and stabbed Nils Sture ten times, then raced headlong out of the castle, calling back to his guards to kill the prisoners, which they did. The king was found wandering alone in the forest that night disguised as a peasant.

Back in Stockholm, Erik recovered, apologized, and paid a fine to the Sture family. But the powerful factions at court, realizing he could slip into total madness at any time, arranged for Johan's release from prison so he would be ready to take the throne at a moment's notice.

Strangely, the death knell of Erik's reign was not his insanity or his stabbing an innocent nobleman. It was marrying beneath him. Having finally given up on winning Elizabeth Tudor or any other royal bride, in the summer of 1567 he secretly married the lovely Karin Mansdotter, a barmaid who had been his mistress since 1565 and had given him a daughter in 1566. Karin came of sturdy peasant stock—just the kind of people Erik trusted—and her father was a jailer. Whatever her humble origins, she was kind and compassionate, and had a way of calming Erik when insanity descended on him. The king, for his part, was deeply in love with her.

By the New Year of 1568, when Karin gave him a son and heir, Erik seemed to be his old self again, though that that wasn't necessarily a good thing. On July 4, Erik publicly married Karin in a lavish royal wedding and then crowned her queen of Sweden. A week later, Erik's many enemies rose up against him, and he surrendered on September 28. Johan took up the reins of government as King Johan III.

Erik and Karin were held in genteel confinement in various palaces. Karin had two sons during her imprisonment who died young. In 1574 Johan released her from prison so that his troublesome brother would have no more legitimate offspring who might one day try to take the throne. Karin was given a royal estate where she lived beloved by her tenants until her death in 1612 at the age of sixty-one.

Erik, however, was a source of constant worry to the new king. Over the years, Johan discovered numerous plots to free and reinstate him. On more than one occasion, Erik himself tried to escape. In 1572, Johan made Erik's guards swear an oath that they would kill Erik if they caught him trying to escape again. The king sent suggestions to Erik's jailers on ways to kill him: smother him with a feather pillow, bleed him ostensibly for health reasons but take too much blood, and poison him with opium or arsenic. In February 1577, the king learned of yet another conspiracy to free Erik and hand him back the throne. Apparently, King Johan had had enough.

It seems that Johan carefully planned the poisoning. In the case of a royal illness, protocol demanded that a team of doctors—as many as a dozen—assist the patient, confer and consult with one another, and write copious notes on symptoms and treatment. But the official report on Erik's final illness was written by two priests in the vaguest of terms. Erik had been sick for years, they said, complaining of pain in his chest and stomach. After feeling ill for several days, they reported, he received Holy Communion, lay quietly, and died at two o'clock on the morning of February 26. This illness does not sound at all like the vomit-spewing, sheet-soiling, shrieking-in-agony symptoms of arsenic poisoning.

Royal corpses, especially those suspected of having died of poison, were invariably autopsied in front of numerous physicians and noble witnesses. Not Erik's. Philip Kern, King Johan's valet, performed a hasty embalming, which was followed by a perfunctory funeral and a burial without the pomp and circumstance due a king.

MODERN POSTMORTEM AND DIAGNOSIS

In 1958, Professor Carl-Herman Hjorstjö of the University of Lund began an investigation to determine if Erik had been poisoned. His team found the king's remains in a black shroud, black cap, and black velvet shoes. The mad monarch had had excellent teeth—all thirty-two remained at death, with only two decayed. He had stood about five foot nine.

Researchers quickly determined that Philip Kern had had no idea how to embalm a corpse. He simply wrapped everything from the neck down in bandages and smeared on beeswax, which resulted in the loss of most of the fleshy parts of the body. Large amounts of arsenic were found in dried-out clumps of tissue in the king's loin region—what would have been his intestines—and in his left lung, on his scalp (from sweat), in the roots of his hair, and in his nail beds. The other parts of his hair had very little arsenic, proof that it had not been applied after death as part of the embalming process. The embalming material itself, the beeswax, contained almost no arsenic.

The greatest proof of poisoning was discovered in the king's funeral suit. The black velvet should have had 8.2 parts per million of arsenic. But it had more than four times that amount, much of it evidently absorbed from the decomposing body.

Johan III ruled Sweden for twenty-four years. Though suspicious and hot-tempered like his brother, the nobility far preferred him, and no one ever poisoned his pea soup.

12

IVAN IV, the TERRIBLE, CZAR of RUSSIA, 1530–1584; HIS MOTHER, ELENA GLINSKAYA, ca. 1510–1538; and HIS FIRST WIFE, ANASTASIA ROMANOVNA, 1530–1560

On March 15, 1584, the ailing fifty-four-year-old czar Ivan the Terrible of Russia invited the English ambassador to walk with him through his treasure chamber, deep in the heart of the Kremlin fortress. The ambassador gaped at the golden goblets, silver plates, rare icons, and loose gemstones. The czar picked up some turquoises, known for their magical properties, and peered at them in the palm of his hand. "See how they change color," he said. "They turn pale, they announce my death, I am poisoned."

He pointed out his most valuable possession of all—his unicorn horn—which had cost him the enormous sum of 70,000 rubles. Ivan instructed his doctors to draw a circle on a table with the tip of the unicorn horn, and he had servants bring him spiders and place them on the table. The spiders that crawled away lived, but those that entered the unicorn circle died at once. "That is a sure sign," he said, "the unicorn horn can no longer save me." Poison, he believed, had killed his mother and his beloved first wife. Now it was his turn. Panic-stricken that he had been poisoned by a brew so toxic even his unicorn horn proved fruitless, he fainted, and two days later he was dead. Centuries later, Russian scientists would find poison in the exhumed remains of the czar, his mother, and his wife.

Ivan was the longed-for son and heir of Grand Prince Vasily III of Muscovy, the Russian principality that, after centuries of warfare, had gobbled up its neighbors and centralized power. Ivan's mother—the czar's younger, second wife—was the scintillating, red-haired Elena Glinskaya, daughter of a Lithuanian refugee. After four years of marriage, on August 25, 1530, just as her first child, Ivan, was slipping into the light of day, thunder rattled the Kremlin and lightning struck a turret. It was an omen of things to come.

When Ivan was three, his father died of a massive infection, leaving Elena regent, served by a council of her relatives and her reputed lover. The nobles, called boyars, were not pleased. Russia needed a strong warrior for a ruler, they believed, not a small child, a foreign woman, her lover, and her rapacious family.

Aware of their antagonism, within days of her husband's death the shrewd Elena imprisoned her opponents, hanging dozens, beating and starving others. Despite her gender and her youth, she achieved much for Russia in a short time and defended it against rampaging Tatars, Kazaks, and Poles. She reformed the currency, signed an armistice to end hostilities with the king of Lithuania, and concluded a treaty with Sweden for free trade.

The effectiveness of a young female regent further outraged the boyars who fought her every move. To check their power, Elena passed laws to limit the amount of land they could hold and increased their taxes. Many boyars wanted her dead. Perhaps it came as no surprise when, after five years of rule, on April 3, 1538, Elena was seized with horrible stomach pains and died soon after at about the age of twenty-eight. No one doubted she had been poisoned. Certainly her eight-year-old son, Ivan, didn't.

The boyars' reaction to her death was immediate and violent. They imprisoned and executed her supporters, then started fighting among themselves for dominance. Frequently, young Ivan witnessed courtiers and servants being dragged away to their deaths. People were stabbed, strangled, drowned, hanged, beheaded, ripped apart by starving hunting dogs, and flayed alive.

Throughout the years of feuding, no one seemed to notice that Ivan was becoming weird. He tortured and killed animals. He cut them open, stabbed their eyes, and hurled puppies off the Kremlin ramparts. He listened to their howls of agony as if they were music. Perhaps he imagined the animals were the boyars who had poisoned his mother and ruined his life. In between his torture sessions, Ivan read the Bible and prostrated himself so much that he developed a callus on his forehead.

At sixteen, Ivan took power and had himself crowned czar—the Russian term for "Caesar," and a grander appellation than a mere grand prince. Czar Ivan IV had reached his full height, which a twentieth-century examination of his bones proved to be six feet. He was slender, with a hawk nose, piercing blue eyes, and long reddish-brown hair and beard. Even at that age, he drank more than was good for him.

It is a truth universally acknowledged that a single czar in possession of a good fortune must be in want of a czarina. Ivan held a *smotriny*, a kind of Russian marriage beauty pageant, the winner of which would become czarina. He sent judges throughout all his lands to examine marriageable girls, rejecting those with acne, bad breath, ill health, crooked teeth, a limp, or a squint. A few dozen finalists arrived in Moscow, where midwives poked them to make sure they were virgins. Out of this group, Ivan chose Anastasia Romanovna, a beautiful brunette from an ancient noble family. At first, Ivan liked her gentleness, piety, and modesty, but he quickly fell in love with her. They married on February 3, 1547, and though he was never faithful to her, his love for her was clear to all.

The young czar was an energetic, ambitious ruler. He rebuilt Moscow after the Great Fire of 1547, revised the law code, created the first parliament, and introduced the first printing press. Militarily ambitious, he led armies to conquer the Khanates of Kazan in the east and Astrakhan in the south along the Caspian Sea. In 1558, he conquered the Baltic port of Narva, in what is now Estonia, and started trading directly with England. He diluted the power of the boyars—whom he never forgave for poisoning his mother—by allowing commoners to compete for top positions in the military and government. Anastasia encouraged him in making sure that merit, not birth, resulted in promotion. Ivan's most lasting contribution, visible to anyone in Red Square today, was St. Basil's Cathedral, a flamboyant medley of eight asymmetrical cupolas, each capped by a different-shaped, brightly colored onion dome.

The czar was immensely popular with his people. The English ambassador wrote, "He uses great familiarity, as well unto all his nobles and subjects, as also unto strangers, which serve him in his wars or in occupations. And by this means he is not only beloved of his nobles and commons, but also held in great dread and fear through all his dominions, so that I think no prince in Christendom is more feared of his own than he is, nor yet better beloved."

With Anastasia by his side, Ivan IV governed the country with relative wisdom and calm. But she grew weaker from each successive pregnancy—six in nine years, though only two sons, Ivan, born in 1554, and Feodor, born in 1557, survived. It is possible her body was not able to produce enough red blood cells to sustain her pregnancies, resulting in iron-deficiency anemia. Symptoms include exhaustion, headaches, shortness of breath, and a compromised immune system that allows other illnesses to take root. After a serious monthlong illness, Czarina Anastasia died on August 7, 1560, at about the age of thirty.

With the loss of Anastasia, madness gripped Ivan's soul. Paranoia devoured him. Despite his wife's deteriorating health over a period of many months, if not years, he was convinced his nobles had murdered her. First, they had poisoned his mother. And now his wife. He was going to wreak a terrible revenge.

Ivan the Terrible was born.

Seemingly on a whim, Ivan arrested nobles and palace officials. The lucky ones were exiled to monasteries in harsh climates. The unlucky starved to death in dungeons, or were tortured to death, burned alive, strangled, crushed by millstones, drowned in the river, beheaded, or had their throats cut. The unluckiest of all he slow-roasted on a grill, boiled to death in a cauldron, or impaled on ten-foot wooden stakes through the anus, where they quivered in agony for days until death released them. And Ivan didn't limit his cruelty to the men he believed were plotting against him: he did the same to their families—even young children—and servants.

He created a new group of soldiers called *oprichniki* who terrorized the populace in the czar's name. Sitting on his throne, Ivan enjoyed watching them rape and torture citizens in front of him. Often, he joined in the fun, as did his elder son when he was old enough. One of the czar's favorite games was to set naked women loose in the palace chasing after chickens, while the *oprichniki* shot the women with arrows.

Ivan offered some prisoners a pardon if they killed their close relatives—a sibling, a parent, a child—and then had them executed for murder. Kremlin Square, now known as Red Square, became a reeking slaughterhouse, with gallows, scaffolds, bonfires, and torture implements. Despite his bloodthirstiness, the people of Russia respected Ivan as a great ruler. His mental instability meant he was touched by God himself, who could be equally harsh and unjust.

Though Ivan always mourned the loss of Anastasia, his grief certainly didn't cool his ardor toward women. He had seven more wives. One he reportedly poisoned, another was reportedly poisoned by an unknown enemy, one he had drowned for adultery, three were sent to convents where two of them died under suspicious circumstances, and one survived him.

In 1568, unhappily married to his second wife, Ivan decided he wanted to shut her up in a convent and marry Elizabeth I of England. He instructed the English ambassador, Anthony Jenkinson, to take her a proposal of marriage, which he was certain would be accepted immediately.

We can only imagine the reaction of Elizabeth—who had just gotten rid of that other lunatic suitor, Erik XIV of Sweden—when she learned of Ivan's offer. After having a good laugh, she must have considered the situation carefully. As a commercial nation, England didn't want to lose trade with Russia. Elizabeth, adept at avoiding marriage without alienating foreign nations, played for time. But Ivan was no fool and exploded with rage when she didn't gratefully accept his offer immediately. "Thyself thou art nothing but a vulgar wench," he wrote, "and thou behavest like one! I give up all intercourse with thee. Moscow can do without the English peasants."

In retaliation at Elizabeth for refusing his divine magnificence, Ivan opened the port of Narva to other foreigners, and it was only with difficulty that England resumed trade. As the years passed and Ivan took and executed more wives and killed more of his subjects, Elizabeth must have thanked heaven for her single status. Here was a monarch who made her father, Henry VIII, look positively civilized.

Ivan's son and heir, Prince Ivan, was like him in many ways: intelligent, tall, and sadistic. He had sent his first two wives to convents for barrenness and, at the age of twenty-seven, married Elena Sheremeteva. A few months later, in the fall of 1581, she was pregnant with their first child, and he hoped for a son and heir. But on November 15, Ivan noticed that his daughter-in-law was wearing only a single dress in the winter chill instead of the three required by royal etiquette. Furious at her immodesty—and the threat she posed to his grandchild— he punched her so hard that she fell and miscarried.

When Prince Ivan heard the news, he found his father and angrily berated him. Ivan, who had suspected for some time that his son was conspiring behind his back to take over the throne, beat him several times about the head and shoulders with the staff he always carried. The heir fell to the ground with a huge gaping hole in his temple.

Ivan looked in shock at his bloody staff. Then he threw himself on his unconscious son and roared in anguish. "Wretch that I am, I have killed my son!" he cried. But he hadn't quite killed him, yet. The prince lasted four days, during which time the czar refused to eat or sleep.

After the prince's death, Ivan became more unhinged than ever, wandering the palace at night with a torch, looking for his son. Early in 1584, Ivan's health took a turn for the worse. He was fifty-four but looked decades older. For years, his appearance had been shocking. Cruelty was etched deeply into his craggy face; his flashing blue eyes were wild. He was bald on the top of his head, and long straggly white hair hung down to past his shoulders. Bloated from overeating and alcohol abuse, Ivan also suffered such severe joint pain that he could barely walk and was usually carried around the palace in a litter. In his final months, he lost weight and his body began to swell. His skin peeled in shreds, giving off a terrible stench. Doctors whispered of a "decomposition of the blood" and "corruption of the bowels." But Ivan was sure it was poison.

That day in the treasure chamber, after Ivan fainted from realizing his unicorn horn had stopped protecting him, he was put to bed and improved somewhat over the next three days. On March 18, he got out of bed, dressed, called the palace singers, and sang with them. Then he sat down to play a game of chess with a friend. Suddenly he was so weak he couldn't set the pieces on the squares. The king and queen fell from his hand and rolled on the floor. His head fell on the chessboard, his arms hung limply. Doctors rubbed his body with vodka. But to no avail. Ivan the Terrible was dead.

MODERN POSTMORTEMS AND DIAGNOSES

In 2000, scientists from the Russian Academy of Sciences exhumed the remains of Ivan's mother, Elena Glinskaya, and his first wife, Anastasia Romanovna, from the necropolis of the Archangel Cathedral inside the Kremlin. Tests revealed that Anastasia had ten times the normal level of mercury in her well-preserved, light-brown braid. Mercury was also found in the remains of her shroud and decayed matter at the bottom of her stone sarcophagus. Scientists obtained similar results when analyzing the red hair of Ivan's mother's, Elena Glinskaya. The amount of mercury was not enough to have been used for embalming, which would have been hundreds or even thousands of times the normal level. John of Lancaster, Duke of Bedford, had been embalmed with quicksilver in 1435. When researchers dug him up in 1860, they found puddles of the stuff in his coffin.

If the women had been poisoned with mercury sublimate, they would have sweated it off in their hair in their final hours. But the amount—ten times the normal level—should not necessarily have been fatal; Agnes Sorel had more than ten thousand times the normal amount of mercury in her remains. Considering Anastasia's lingering illness, however, such a small amount may have been enough to tip her over the edge.

Not enough is known about the final illness of Ivan's mother to postulate what killed her. Had she been feeling unwell for months? Could she have died of a ruptured appendix or gastric ulcer? It is possible that both women were given mercury in a medication or used it in a pomade on their hair to prevent lice. Both women had elevated levels of lead, as well, but nothing that could have proved fatal. And, indeed, all the royal women exhumed in the Kremlin vault had high levels of lead, arsenic, and mercury, probably from their cosmetics. Russian women painted their faces to look like dolls, with silvery-white lead, mercury, and arsenic skin, and bright red cinnabar-mercury cheeks.

In 1963, a special commission of the Russian Ministry of Culture opened Ivan's coffin, buried in the Kelmisvi Chapel of the Kremlin, to conduct a forensic analysis of his remains. He had severe arthritis—his cartilage and ligaments had ossified—and must have suffered excruciating pain, which certainly hadn't improved his mood.

Though Ivan believed he was being poisoned, most physicians agree that, despite suffering from various serious illnesses at the time of his death, including possibly cirrhosis of the liver and kidney disease, he was felled by a massive stroke. Researchers discovered only trace amounts of arsenic in his bones, within the normal range. They did, however, find much higher than normal levels of mercury. Scientists have speculated that, given Ivan's sexual voraciousness, he may have had syphilis and received the standard mercury treatment for it, which over time would have caused paranoia and violent mood swings.

Syphilis, however, would not explain his sadism as a child. He must have been born with a psychological disorder, made worse by the early loss of his parents, the almost daily violence he witnessed for many years, and the mercury in his system. Ivan was clearly born terrible, but life—and his medications—made him more so.

13

GRAND DUKE FRANCESCO I de MEDICI of TUSCANY, 1541–1587, and GRAND DUCHESS BIANCA CAPPELLO, 1548–1587

When Grand Duchess Bianca of Tuscany sat down to dinner on the afternoon of October 8, 1587, she must have looked around the glittering banquet with great satisfaction. Once she had been a wanted criminal with a price on her head, chased by bounty hunters, and mired in poverty and disgrace. Now she luxuriated in wealth and power. And she owed it all to the man sitting morosely next to her, forty-six-year-old Grand Duke Francesco I de Medici, dark and plump, with small neat features and a closely trimmed moustache and beard.

This would be their last banquet. Within hours, both would be taken severely ill, and after days of unspeakable torment, both would die. And despite exhumation and state-of-the-art medical tests, controversy rages even today about whether they died naturally or got a bit of help.

Bianca was Francesco's second wife. The daughter of a Venetian nobleman, at the age of fifteen she had become pregnant and eloped to Florence with a swaggering sack of Italian testosterone named Piero Buonaventuri. Even though she married her seducer, her furious family sent bounty hunters to capture and return her so they could wall her up in a convent.

Francesco, the heir to the Tuscan throne, had first seen her sitting at the window of her in-laws' house. He fell in love at first sight with the girl with wide blue eyes, golden-red hair, and flawless white skin, and arranged to see her at the palaces of noble ladies. Her interest in him must have quickened when, in June 1564, Duke Cosimo retired, allowing Francesco to have an equal title and most of the power.

In July 1564, Bianca gave birth to Pellegrina, her daughter with Piero, and sometime after that she became Francesco's mistress. The young duke showered her with property, jewels, and income. Her blatantly unfaithful husband was overjoyed at the opportunity to monetize her. As for Bianca, she went willingly. Though slothful and sullen, the prince was attractive in a swarthy way. At twenty-three, he was seven years her senior. The Venetian ambassador described him as "of low stature, thin, dark complexioned and of a melancholy disposition." "He shows little grace in dress," wrote another ambassador. Quiet and thoughtful, he was "much absorbed by the love of women" and "set little store by virtue," certainly a bonus for Bianca.

In December 1565, Francesco dutifully married the plain, thin-lipped princess his father had picked out for him, Joanna of Austria. Looks aside, it was Joanna's stiff Germanic manner that irritated Francesco the most. With more piety than wit, Joanna was far readier to criticize than smile. She disapproved of Italian liveliness, somberly predicting that everyone was going to hell. Francesco bought Bianca a gracious palazzo near the palace, which he ran to whenever his wife started nagging him, which was often.

Joanna's greatest complaint was, of course, Bianca, the mere sight of whom could send the grand duchess into paroxysms of rage. Once, when the two women's carriages met head-on on a bridge, Joanna tried to have her husband's mistress thrown into the river. The Tuscan people would have loved to witness such a spectacle, as they despised the mistress, too, seeing that a good portion of their taxes went into her bottomless brocade pockets.

Bianca was also despised by Francesco's brother, Cardinal Ferdinando, eight years his junior. No saintly ascetic, Ferdinando was a worldly man and enjoyed to the fullest the many delights of Rome. Handsome, affable, blue-eyed, and rosy-cheeked, he was immune to Bianca's renowned charm and was a hardworking, capable administrator, well respected in the Vatican. In short, the Medici brothers were polar opposites.

While Francesco didn't seem to care much whether he sullied the Medici name, Ferdinando cared very much indeed. He heard that his brother and his mistress were the objects of dirty jokes not only in Tuscany but across Europe, and it drove him crazy. He was also quite fond of his scorned sister-in-law, Joanna.

It seems that early on, Bianca had her sights set on marrying the duke, who became grand duke in 1569 when the pope raised the status of Tuscany. But there were two large obstacles in her way named Piero and Joanna. The Piero problem was taken care of in 1572, when male relatives of his mistress, after warning him several times to leave her alone, cut him down in front of his house with the grand duke's blessing. After Piero's murder, Bianca persuaded her lover to marry her on two conditions: if Joanna died, of course, and if Bianca gave him a son, as only a son could inherit the throne. Joanna had given him six girls, though only three lived, and she was sickly. Every time Bianca received word that the grand duchess had sneezed, her heart must have soared with hope. Still, the Austrian remained vexingly alive.

As far as giving him a son, Bianca had never been able to conceive after Pellegrina's birth. But in 1576, after twelve years of infertility, Bianca adroitly produced a son, Antonio, whom Francesco delightedly acknowledged as his own. Reports indicated, however, that Bianca had only pretended to be pregnant and had had a servant smuggle the baby into her chamber in a laundry basket as she howled in fake pain. Soon after, the servant was mysteriously attacked by bandits while traveling, though she lived long enough to tell the whole story to a priest.

Ferdinando had always been his brother's undisputed heir. Though a cardinal, he had never received priestly ordination, which was believed to bestow a kind of spiritual tattoo that made marriage forever impossible. This sidestepping of the sacrament of ordination was a tradition among churchmen from royal families, in case the male line died out and they would be required to take the crown, marry, and father children. Now, with the birth of Antonio, the cardinal, who had always disliked his brother's mistress, perceived her as a personal threat.

The problem of Antonio faded in May 1577 when Joanna gave birth to a son, Filippo. But in April 1578, after throwing a tantrum about Bianca, Joanna went into premature labor, ruptured her uterus, gave birth to a dead child, and bled to death at the age of thirty-two.

While the people of Tuscany mourned their grand duchess, Bianca was doing a victory dance. She summoned the royal physician, Pietro Cappelli, from Joanna's deathbed and cried with shrill joy, "Give me your hand and rejoice, for now at last I can make your fortune! Last night the grand duke was here and swore on that crucifix to make me his wife!"

In June 1579, Francesco kept his promise, married Bianca, and had her crowned in a lavish ceremony. Cardinal Ferdinando was horrified that a whore wore the crown of Tuscany and all Europe was laughing about it. He placed spies in her service to make sure she didn't smuggle in another child that, unlike Antonio, could be passed off as legitimate. The situation became more serious in March 1582, when Francesco's heir, four-year-old Don Filippo, died of an illness.

At this point, Francesco should have simply acknowledged his brother as his heir. But Francesco, at Bianca's goading, declared Antonio his heir. Then, in an effort at reconciliation, he invited his brother to go hunting with him at the villa of Poggia a Caiano, outside Florence. The cardinal arrived on September 25, 1587, and was warmly welcomed by Francesco and Bianca.

Francesco apologized for his former harshness, and Ferdinando begged pardon for any seeming disloyalty. Over the next two weeks, as Bianca played the most gracious hostess, the party feasted, played cards, and listened to music. But their favorite pastime was hunting in the swampy area where Francesco had laid out rice paddies. All was seeming harmony, except that Bianca and Ferdinando watched each other like hawks.

On the afternoon of October 8, Francesco and Bianca must have given a typical Renaissance feast. Francesco, brooding and taciturn, slouched in his chair watching servants shoulder enormous platters of traditional dishes such as roasted peacocks with their feathers sewn back on, larded porcupines stuck with cloves, and guinea pigs with French mustard. He had thrown up the past couple of days and still felt queasy, with sharp pains in his stomach. Bianca, overseeing the festivities, was starting to shiver in the hot, crowded banquet hall.

Francesco shook off his symptoms and played cards. He went briefly to his room to drink a healing potion of bezoar stone in broth, then returned to the card room. Two hours after sunset, he began to feel deathly ill, retired, and called his physicians. They diagnosed a fever and put him to bed. Bianca, too, had taken to her bed with fever, diarrhea, and vomiting, though less severe than her husband's. Her main concern was for Francesco, and she was upset she couldn't nurse him. As a result, Cardinal Ferdinando took charge of both sickrooms, working with the physicians and issuing reports about the grand ducal couple's health.

While royal physicians recorded Francesco's symptoms in great detail, they made less mention of Bianca's, merely indicating that her illness was similar to his, if less alarming. Over the following days, Francesco's fever increased, along with copious sweating, vomiting, diarrhea, abdominal pain, and unquenchable thirst. He had difficulty urinating and breathing. Naturally, his physicians bled him almost dry, and gave him pukes (medications to make him vomit) and purges (medications to give him violent blasts of diarrhea), which, unsurprisingly, only worsened his symptoms.

On the morning of Monday, October 19, Francesco began having convulsions. Realizing he was dying, he asked to confess and be given Last Rites. He spoke at length to Ferdinando of matters of state, named eleven-year-old Antonio as his successor, and asked the cardinal to take care of Bianca. Ferdinando promised him he would. For fourteen hours after that, Francesco suffered excruciating pain. He rolled about on the bed screaming so loudly people could hear him several rooms away. Finally, four hours after sunset, Francesco died. The cardinal rode off to Florence to arrange for his brother's funeral and take control of the duchy's treasury and defenses.

Bianca's condition had worsened over the past few days, and she seems to have given up all hope when she realized her husband and protector was dead. Life for her under the vengeful rule of Cardinal Ferdinando, she knew, would prove very difficult indeed. She groaned, "And now I die with my Lord!" And did, eleven hours after Francesco, on the morning of October 20. Naturally, no one thought about giving the crown to an illegitimate changeling child, no matter what the late grand duke had ordered. His wishes in the matter died with him. Polished, capable, thirty-eight-year-old Cardinal Ferdinando would be the new ruler.

CONTEMPORARY POSTMORTEMS

To quash rumors already taking wing that he had poisoned Francesco and Bianca to grab the throne for himself, Ferdinando commanded that both be autopsied before a large crowd, including several doctors, courtiers, and Bianca's twenty-three-year-old daughter. Francesco's autopsy revealed an inflamed, dark-colored liver so hard the surgeons could barely cut it, and a diseased stomach, lungs, and kidneys. The grand duchess had consumption of the lungs (tuberculosis), a diseased liver and uterus, and edema throughout her body—water retention due to a heart, kidney, or liver condition that swelled her limbs.

Clearly, both had been unhealthy well before their final illnesses. Most of the physicians present agreed that the two had died of a tertian fever—what we now call malaria—with no sign of poison. But we must consider that only a brave man would tell the new grand duke, who had been in charge of the sickrooms, that *someone* had murdered his brother.

Two of the physicians, however, were very brave indeed. They believed that the velvety red congestion of Francesco's stomach indicated arsenic poisoning. According to the autopsy report, "The colour of the stomach was red, as it is in inflamed parts, and it occupied a great part of the stomach, being more intense and more reddened in the middle." They "found in them the same kind of poison that had eaten up their internal organs." But these two were overruled. The official verdict was tertian fever.

While it is understandable that sixteenth-century physicians disagreed on the cause of death, it is more surprising that twenty-first century scientists still do as well. Two groups of Italian researchers vehemently disagree on whether the couple died of malaria or arsenic.

After the autopsies, the two corpses went their different ways. Ferdinando gave Francesco a lavish funeral and buried him in the family crypt in the Basilica of San Lorenzo in Florence, next to the unloved Joanna. When questioned whether Bianca should wear the crown in her coffin, he snapped that she had already worn it far too long. When asked where she should be buried, he said, "Wherever you choose, but we will not have her amongst us."

Bianca's body was dumped in an unmarked grave, reportedly in the churchyard just outside San Lorenzo. In 1902, workmen building a new courtyard entrance found a late sixteenth-century coffin by itself, set well apart from the family plots, with no brass plate identifying it. They cracked it open and gazed upon the remains of a woman with thick blond braids and a plain robe. The priest believed it to be Bianca and, startled at having such a fallen woman in his church, hid the body. Recently, researchers have done their best to locate it, but in vain.

Nor has Francesco been allowed to rest in peace. His first exhumation in 1857 found him mummified, a condition that had possibly been caused by extreme dehydration due to eleven days of constant vomiting and diarrhea. Starting in 1945, an anthropologist named Giuseppe Genna began a decadelong study on twenty-three Medici corpses, including Francesco's, to bolster his belief that the shape of an individual's skull determined intelligence, personality, and other traits. In 1947 Genna stripped off the flesh, muscle, and hair to make casts of the Medici skulls. Francesco was reduced to a jumble of brown bones.

MODERN POSTMORTEM AND DUELING DIAGNOSES

In 2004, a team of researchers led by Dr. Gino Fornaciari of the University of Pisa opened up several Medici graves, including Francesco's, and removed small fragments of his femur bone for testing. They also found a dime-sized flake of crusty white skin shaped like Australia, with several long black hairs protruding, all that remained after the 1947 scrubbing.

The team discovered evidence of *Plasmodium falciparum*, the most lethal kind of malaria, in Francesco's bones. This finding, however, doesn't prove that he died of it; he could have had it years earlier. They then tested the material for arsenic. Interestingly, Francesco's bones contained almost no arsenic, despite the grand duke's obsessive, decades-long fiddling with poisons in his palace lab. But a heaping dose of arsenic that killed the grand duke in eleven days would not have had time to show up in bone. The best place to find proof of arsenic poisoning would be in the digestive organs.

It was customary for the organs of the royal dead to be removed, put in pots, and interred in a church other than the one the body was buried in, thereby spreading the honor to more than one church. For centuries, no one knew where Francesco's organs were. Then, in 2005, University of Florence medical history professor Donatella Lippi—who had been part of Dr. Fornaciari's team the year before—found among church records a document that stated that Francesco and Bianca's "viscera were brought to Santa Maria a Bonistallo [a church near the hunting lodge where they died] in four jars."

Crawling around beneath the church, Professor Lippi and her team found the four broken pots with no names on them, but two crucifixes indicated that they contained the organs of two individuals. Scientists took three samples of the thick, crumbly mush inside. Sample A came from a man's liver, but scientists could not determine what organs samples B and C came from, though B was female and C male.

To determine that at least some of the male mush in the pots belonged to Francesco, the team compared the DNA of the male material from the pots with the hair and skin fragment found in Francesco's coffin. They determined that there was a high probability that the material from the pot and the hair/skin fragment belonged to the same individual. The researchers could perform no DNA comparison on the female material, as Bianca's grave has not been found. But if the male material does, indeed, belong to Francesco, then the female remains must be Bianca's.

Additionally, they performed tests to determine the presence of arsenic. All soft tissue samples—A, B, and C—had levels significantly higher than normal. Professor Lippi tested the soil upon which the pots rested and found only trace amounts of arsenic, proving the poison did not enter the pots through contamination.

Some evidence points to the possibility of poisoning. Arsenic symptoms include nausea, nonstop vomiting, cold sweats, unquenchable thirst, the kind of unbearable abdominal pain that had Francesco screaming for fourteen hours, delirium, and restlessness. Francesco's autopsy, too, showed possible signs of arsenic in the inflamed stomach. Furthermore, it would be unusual for two people suffering from malaria to come down with violent symptoms at the same time and die within hours of each other. *Plasmodium falciparum* incubates nine to fourteen days after an infected mosquito bite, and those with malaria had a range of reactions depending on their genetics, their immune systems, and their overall health. Some victims recovered completely. If a group was infected at the same time, those who died usually did so many days apart. For instance, in 1562, when Francesco's mother and two brothers came down with malaria, one died November 20, another December 6, and the third December 17.

Dr. Fornaciari, however, strongly believes the couple died of malaria and that the DNA test is unreliable, as Francesco's bones had been scrubbed clean. The skin fragment must be the result of contamination during the exhumation process, and indications of a genetic match are thus incorrect. He also believes that Francesco's organs were never in the pots, which seemed to him to be from the nineteenth century rather than the sixteenth. In the nineteenth century—but not the sixteenth—arsenic was used in the embalming process, which would explain the arsenic found in the mush.

Professor Lippi, on the other hand, maintains that the skin fragment is Francesco's and has consulted experts who agree that the pots are indeed from the late sixteenth century. She believes the amount of arsenic in the pots was not nearly enough to embalm but was certainly sufficient to kill over a period of a few days.

As for Bianca and Francesco's symptoms, the most telling sign of malaria is high fever, which both suffered. Arsenic poisoning does not cause fever and usually kills its victims in two or three days, not eleven. So it is quite likely that both had malaria, though initially Bianca didn't seem to have a serious case, and Francesco at one point seemed to be recovering. Perhaps Cardinal Ferdinando used the opportunity to prevent their recovery by adding a bit of poison to their medications, which were not tested by tasters. Francesco's fourteen hours of screaming at the top of his lungs shortly before he died might have been the result of spiked medicine.

Despite the shadow of murder that always hung over him—and still does, despite modern science—Ferdinando had a successful reign of twenty-two years, during which his skilled management burnished Tuscany's tarnished image. He boosted commerce and industry, supported the arts, reduced taxation, and crafted a fairer justice system. He established Medici banks across Europe and issued an edict of tolerance for Jews and Protestants. In 1589, having handed his red hat back to the pope, he married a French princess, Christine of Lorraine, and, making up for lost time, fathered nine children in quick succession.

He was a kind uncle to Antonio, arranging an excellent education for him and giving him large incomes and grand estates. But Grand Duke Ferdinando never forgave Bianca. He removed all her portraits and coats of arms from the Medici palaces and replaced them with those of Joanna of Austria. Though the cause of the deaths of Francesco and Bianca remains in doubt, Ferdinando's hatred is as clear as day.

14

GABRIELLE d'ESTRÉES, MISTRESS of KING HENRI IV of FRANCE, 1573–1599

On Thursday, April 8, 1599, twenty-six-year-old Gabrielle d'Estrées, duchesse of Beaufort, entered Paris for a festive weekend that would culminate in her wedding to King Henri IV and her coronation as queen of France on Easter Sunday, three days later. The people of Paris rejoiced. The match was a true love story, and their beloved Gabrielle's diplomatic skill and insightful advice had played a major role in ending the religious civil wars that had devastated France for more than thirty years. Parisians have always been captivated by beauty, and their new queen would be the most ravishing in the world—tall and voluptuous, with pale blond hair and wide blue eyes.

But many in the higher echelons of society opposed the wedding. Gabrielle wasn't exactly a virgin princess. In fact, she had been the king's mistress for eight years—while he was still married to Marguerite de Valois, whom he had locked up in a castle—had given him three children, and was six months pregnant with the fourth. Her enemies—and there were many—felt the king's marriage to a harlot shamed all of France, confused the royal succession (which son would inherit the throne: the eldest who was technically a bastard, or the one born after the wedding?), and squandered a valuable opportunity for a political alliance with a foreign country.

Within hours, Gabrielle would become not a queen but a corpse, and given the timing, everyone assumed she had been poisoned.

The daughter of Antoine d'Estrées, marquis de Coevres, Gabrielle grew up in turbulent times. The Catholic French king Henri III battled the Catholic League—a union of Spain, the pope, and the Jesuits angered by his leniency with heretics. The league was especially dismayed that the king's heir was none other than the wisecracking heretic-in-chief, King Henri of Navarre, who had converted to Catholicism after the Saint Bartholomew's Day Massacre in 1572 and then abjured it as soon as he escaped. The league grew more insistent on regime change in 1589, when Henri III was stabbed to death by a fanatical monk, making the heretic-in-chief now king of France.

When Henri IV visited Coevres Castle in 1590, he fell in love at first sight with the gorgeous seventeen-year-old daughter of the house. The feeling was not mutual. Gabrielle was already having an affair with Henri's friend, the dashing duc de Bellegarde. And Henri, twenty years her senior, was no Adonis with his big nose, bowlegs, and ragged clothing. Although he was the king of France, his prospects of clinging to the throne and uniting the country were quite slim, considering the superpowers lined up against him.

The king told the duc de Bellegarde to find another mistress and continued to pursue Gabrielle, showing up periodically at her father's castle. The marquis was outraged at the scandal; not only would his daughter be known across France as a fallen woman, she would also be an adulteress: the king was a married man. In 1592, he forced his daughter to wed an obese, elderly widower, the Sieur d'Amerval, who was "ill-endowed as to graces of person and of mind," according to her brother. Gabrielle's sister and aunt reported that she spent every day of her marriage weeping until, three months later, Henri freed himself from battle long enough to spirit her away from her husband.

Soon Gabrielle realized that Henri was, in fact, dazzlingly attractive for his vivacious wit, good nature, boundless energy, and penetrating intellect, and fell deeply in love with him. She insisted on following him on campaign where she lived in cold, drafty tents, washed his clothes, and made sure he had a hot dinner after a day's fighting. When he took the field, she remained in their tent writing his political and diplomatic dispatches. In the evening, they would discuss the events of the day.

Henri wrote, "Last evening I found three bullet holes burned into the fabric of my mistress' tent, and begged her to go to her house in Paris, where her life would not be endangered, but she laughed and was deaf to my pleas . . . She replied that only in my presence is she pleased. I entertain no fears for myself, but daily tremble for her."

In 1593, Gabrielle saw all too clearly that the political, religious, and military stalemate paralyzing France—and preventing Henri from being acknowledged king by large segments of the Catholic population—could go on for years. She convinced Henri that if he converted—again—almost all Frenchmen would prefer him to Spanish King Philip II. Shrugging, Henri reportedly declared, "Paris is well worth a Mass." Paris opened its gates and Henri was finally crowned.

Although the civil war was over, tensions between Catholics and Protestants continued, often flaring up into murders and riots. Henri wanted to craft an edict that spelled out the rights of Huguenots in France. Henri's sister Catherine of Navarre, a rigid Protestant like her mother, the late Queen Jeanne of Navarre, set to work on the Huguenots, and Gabrielle, a Catholic, set to work on the Catholics.

One by one, Gabrielle persuaded powerful Catholic families to accept the king's edict of religious toleration. Henri wrote, "My mistress has become an orator of unequaled excellence, so fiercely does she argue the cause of the new Edict." In 1598, the Edict of Nantes granted Huguenots certain limited rights, a true compromise, as Catholics didn't want them to have any at all. Henri knew his people would never have accepted the edict without Gabrielle's diplomatic skill.

In 1596, Henri appointed her to the royal council, a shocking honor for a woman, and a fallen one at that. He softened the blow by naming his puritanical sister Catherine, as well. Gabrielle's brother wrote, "My sister was more powerful than the king at this time, His Majesty's faith in her being so great that he left in her hands many matters that otherwise would have required his personal attention."

But Gabrielle hoped for something more than wealth and power. She wanted to marry Henri. She, at least, had obtained a divorce in 1594 with a little pressure from the king, who badgered her husband to swear he had never consummated the marriage. With the country stabilized, Henri realized he needed to remarry and sire heirs. If he died without a legitimate son, France would once again explode in civil war.

Foreign rulers eagerly proffered their daughters and nieces, but Henri, after pretending to consider them and studying flattering portraits, rejected them all. He told his advisers he wanted a wife who was beautiful, good-natured, and able to bear children, clearly referring to Gabrielle as none of the virgin princesses on the market had ever borne a child.

But before he could marry, he needed to divorce Marguerite, who had been imprisoned in a distant castle for many years for having sex with gardeners and stable boys. Marguerite, knowing Henri could do a Henry VIII on her—that is, behead her for adultery—agreed that the marriage was invalid because she had been forced to marry him against her will. And, indeed, at the wedding ceremony, when she refused to say *I do*, her brother, King Charles IX of France, had been seen angrily pushing her head up and down in a forced nod.

The pope, recognizing the difficulty Henri was in, was willing to grant a divorce, as long as the king promised to marry Marie de Medici, daughter of the late Francesco I de Medici and Joanna of Austria and niece of the ruling grand duke, Ferdinando. But Henri, aside from wanting to marry Gabrielle, was repelled at marrying into the family of French queen mother Catherine de Medici, who had tried to murder him on Saint Bartholomew's Day.

After waiting years for the annulment, finally, on March 2, 1599, Henri shrugged it off and announced the wedding would take place on April 11, Easter Sunday. In front of the entire French court, he held up his diamond coronation ring and presented it to Gabrielle as an engagement ring. Gabrielle's wildest ambitions were about to be realized.

Still, something was off. Though she had sailed through her three previous pregnancies in glowing health, she didn't feel well with this one. She had trouble sleeping, and when she did, she had horrific nightmares, waking more exhausted than when she had gone to bed. The woman known for her cheerful vitality was suddenly depressed and irritable.

Henri had decided that, given the holiness of the Easter holiday, they would not live in sin for three days before the wedding. He would stay at the palace of Fontainebleau, outside Paris, and she would travel by barge to the capital to enjoy the celebrations. They would meet at the altar on Sunday. When Henri bid her farewell on the bank of the river, she burst into tears and clung to him as if she thought she would never see him again. He comforted her and sent her on her way, chalking her emotions up to pregnancy combined with wedding jitters.

In Paris, Gabrielle and her ladies lodged with a good friend of the king's, the Italian banker Sebastian Zamet. But after eating a sumptuous meal that included a lemon, she suddenly felt sick with nausea, dizziness, headache, and stabbing pains in her stomach. She canceled her appearance at several gala events but decided she was well enough to attend a service at a nearby church. Once seated for the service, however, she fainted several times. Her servants put her in a litter and carried her back to Zamet's, where she walked in the garden to revive herself. There she was seized with an "apoplectic fit," according to witnesses.

Fearing that Zamet had poisoned her—he was Italian, after all—she insisted that she and her entourage move to her aunt's house, where she was put to bed. No sooner had Gabrielle slipped between the sheets than she had "thick succeeding convulsions," according to Henri's finance minister, the duc de Sully, "so dreadful as amazed all that were present, and in a word all the symptoms of approaching death . . . New convulsions turned her black and disfigured her so horribly," he continued, and she suffered "agonies that left her hardly anything of human in her figure." When Gabrielle opened her eyes, she said she was blind. Looking at the grotesque form writhing uncontrollably on the bed, some of her ladies-in-waiting fainted.

One royal physician named La Rivière "came in great haste upon this occasion," wrote Henri's contemporary, the chronicler Agrippa d'Aubigné, "with others of the king's physicians, and entering but three steps into her chamber, when he saw the extraordinary condition she was in, went away, saying to his brother physicians, 'This is the hand of God.'"

Gabrielle had gone into labor three months early. The physicians hoped that if they delivered the child, she might recover. They tore the child out in pieces, bled her, and gave her four enemas to remove the afterbirth, but it remained firmly wedged in her womb. By six in the evening on Friday, April 9, Gabrielle had fallen into a coma. The physicians placed smelling salts under her nose and burned feathers an inch away from the soles of her feet, but nothing could rouse her. At five o'clock on Saturday morning, April 10, Gabrielle d'Estrées died, thirty-six hours before she would have been crowned queen of France.

The timing of Gabrielle's death was so strange that naturally rumors of poison swept across Europe. The likely culprits were the Vatican or the House of Medici, which had been violently opposed to Henri's marriage to Gabrielle and hoped he would marry Marie de Medici instead. Grand Duke Ferdinando de Medici was already reputed to have poisoned his brother Francesco and his sister-in-law Bianca. His reputation as a poisoner was not unwarranted, as his correspondence in the Medici Archives proves he indeed made attempts to poison political enemies. But it wasn't just the Italians who were suspect; many important Frenchmen had railed against having a whore as queen, embarrassing the entire nation.

Gabrielle had died grimacing in agony. Her ladies, trying to rearrange her face for the funeral, could not coax her grotesquely twisted features back into place, which added to the belief of poison. The coffin was closed at the funeral.

CONTEMPORARY POSTMORTEM

Henri's physicians and surgeons conducted an autopsy and announced that they found "a lung and the liver corrupt, a kidney stone and an injury to the brain." Kidney stone aside, the other changes could have been postmortem or, especially in the case of the brain hemorrhage, could have been the result of her final illness rather than the cause of it. They found nothing unusual in her digestive tract, but blamed her death on "a corrupt lemon," the fumes of which had risen to her brain, killing her. The Tuscan ambassador to France reported in his dispatch of April 17, "The body was opened. One could not discover the least indication from which one could deduce any suspicion of poison."

After the funeral, Gabrielle's effigy was placed in a small chamber in the king's private apartments in the Louvre and dressed in a new gown daily. Henri wrote, "The root of my love is dead; it will not spring up again." He visited the figure for many years, even after he had caved in to the pope's wishes and married Marie de Medici and, perhaps as a protest, taken the first in a series of nubile young mistresses. Despite the king's genuine sadness at the loss of Gabrielle, the root of his love continued to spring up until his dying day. In fact, Henri had fifty-six known mistresses. But he was faithful only to Gabrielle.

MODERN DIAGNOSIS

Though Gabrielle's body was destroyed in the French Revolution, today's doctors are fairly certain as to what caused her death: eclampsia, a disorder usually presenting in the second half of pregnancy caused by high blood pressure and organ dysfunction. Her symptoms fit exactly with those of eclampsia: nausea, vomiting, vertigo, abdominal pain, convulsions, blindness, coma, organ failure, and death.

15

TYCHO BRAHE, ASTRONOMER
and IMPERIAL MATHEMATICIAN,
1546–1601

When the world's greatest astronomer, the colorful Tycho Brahe, sat down to a hearty banquet at a neighboring nobleman's house in Prague on October 13, 1601, he must have looked forward to a convivial night of wine, food, charming women, and witty conversation, all of which this fun-loving Dane enjoyed in great measure. Hobnobbing with the rich and powerful was part of his job as imperial mathematician to Holy Roman Emperor Rudolf II, and Brahe did it— as he did everything—with great gusto.

Brahe's astonishing intellect made him a favorite banquet guest. For forty years, he had spent the wee hours of the night recording extraordinarily precise observations of the planets and stars with cunning instruments of his own devising. While we often refer to a genius as an Einstein, back then people would call one a Brahe.

Moreover, Brahe was a jolly soul with an eccentric, extroverted personality. Known to his contemporaries as a "man of easy fellowship," he "did not hold anger and offense, but was ever ready to forgive." Redhaired, blue-eyed, and sporting a trim pointed beard and handlebar moustache, the astronomer wore a metal nose reported to be either gold or silver, as he had lost the bridge of his nose at the age of twenty in a duel over a mathematical formula. When the glue holding his nose in place came loose, he would remove the prosthesis, take a bottle of glue out of his pocket, and glue it back on.

Brahe's eccentricities were widely known. He had a dwarf jester named Jepp with supposed psychic abilities who sat under his dining room table during meals. For years, Brahe kept a beer-swigging pet elk in his castle. One night the elk drank too much beer, fell down a staircase, and died. It is not known if Jepp predicted this.

Noble banquets offered delicious food, fine wine, beautiful music, a glittering table, and fascinating conversation. But there was one downside. They went on for hours, during which time guests were expected to eat and drink until they nearly popped. It was bad etiquette to excuse yourself to use a chamber pot. Brahe's assistant, the contentious twenty-nine-year-old Johannes Kepler, so loathed boring, bladder-bursting banquets that he wrote into his employment contract with Brahe that he would not be expected to attend them.

As candlelight flickered on golden cups and silver plates and laughter wafted around him, Brahe felt increasing abdominal discomfort. He must have thought he would be fine once he got home, which was just across the street. After all, the robust fifty-four-year-old Dane had never known any serious illness in his life.

By the time he arrived home, the need to relieve his bladder was agonizing. Grunting with relief he dropped his britches and . . . nothing. Not a drop. And so began a four-hundred-year-old mystery involving rumors of poison, theories of natural illness, and dueling scientific analyses of a skeleton with a red walrus moustache and damage to the bridge of its nose.

At fourteen, Brahe witnessed a solar eclipse that changed his life; he decided to become an astronomer. His proud noble family, hoping he would win titles and honors at court or in the military, looked down on his choice. But years later Brahe wrote to a friend, "Let others compliment themselves on their high birth and look for honor in the deeds of their ancestors . . . For myself I aspire to higher things . . . For there are few, very few, whom God lets see what is high above us."

At the time, to predict eclipses, conjunctions, and other heavenly events, astronomers used the Ptolemaic Tables, composed in the sec-

ond century ad by the Egyptian Claudius Ptolemy, and the Copernican
Tables, created by the early sixteenth-century astronomer Nicolaus
Copernicus. In 1563, at the tender age of seventeen, Brahe observed a
conjunction of Jupiter and Saturn and realized that both tables used to
predict the event were incorrect.

This wasn't news. In the early fifteenth century, a naval captain exploring for Prince Henry the Navigator of Portugal reported his difficulty in mapping his course with the current tables, stating, "With all
due respect to the renowned Ptolemy, we found everything the oppo-
site of what he said." The most serious concern was that astronomical
miscalculations doomed the accuracy of horoscopes, which kings and
emperors relied upon for political and military decisions.

Brahe, young as he was, realized that any true progress in the fields
of astronomy and its sister science, astrology, must be based on accurate observations, night after night, for many years. He bought a
radius—an instrument similar to a large compass that could measure
the angles of the stars and planets—and spent his nights recording
his observations. Over time, he invented his own instruments to better
measure the distances between planetary bodies. Brahe's decades of
records, made with the naked eye—Galileo wouldn't invent the tele-
scope until 1610—became the largest collection of astronomical observations ever made until then.

In Brahe's time, scientists endeavored to fit their observations—often
fudging them a great deal—into the dogma of established theory. For
instance, astronomers believed the planets had a perfectly circular orbit around the sun because a circle was divine geometry, flawless and
permanent, like the Creator of the universe itself. Any other view was
considered not just incorrect, but blasphemous.

In 1572, Brahe observed a very bright new star in the constellation
Cassiopeia. Since antiquity, theory maintained that the universe beyond the moon's orbit was immutable and eternal, and changes could
occur only between the moon and the earth. There was, it was believed,
simply no such thing as a new or dying star. The Bible said God had
created the heavens at the beginning of time; it didn't say he was still
creating them. Therefore, the new object had to be something located
below the orbit of the moon. Brahe easily proved otherwise with his

nightly observations, shattering two thousand years of astronomical theory. His 1573 book *De nova stella* called his many critics "thick wits" and "blind watchers of the sky."

With his unconventional approach to science—making theory fit observation, rather than the other way around—Brahe broke the bonds of fossilized thought. Though his fame spread across Europe, his Tychonic view of the solar system was faulty. He correctly believed the moon orbited the earth, and the planets revolved around the sun, but incorrectly believed the sun orbited the earth.

For twenty-one years, Brahe conducted astronomical and alchemical research in a castle of his own design, Uraniborg, funded by King Frederick II of Denmark. He established it as a renowned scientific center. Kings, queens, nobles, and scholars from across Europe visited to see the marvel and meet the man known as one of the most brilliant in the world. But when King Frederick's nineteen-year-old son, Christian IV, came to power in 1597, he exiled Brahe, reportedly for having an affair with his mother, Queen Sophie. Brahe found a haven in Prague, at the court of Holy Roman Emperor Rudolph II, where he became the official imperial astronomer and mathematician. The emperor hoped Brahe's astronomical research would result in more accurate horoscopes. Brahe, however, had long ago decided that astrology could not produce accurate predictions—two astrologers using the same exact data often came up with diametrically opposed prognostications. But he used his position to calm the agitated monarch, who was steadily slipping into mental illness, and to buoy him up from debilitating depression.

In February 1600, Brahe hired a new assistant, a twenty-eight-year-old German named Johannes Kepler. Though he was an excellent mathematician, Kepler suffered severe hypochondria and violent mood swings. He had published a book in which he laid out his own astronomical theory—that the universe itself was an image of God, with the Sun corresponding to the Father, the stellar sphere to the Son, and the intervening space to the Holy Ghost. Kepler took the position with Brahe to obtain access to his employer's forty years of observations to prove his own theories. He couldn't make his own observations; smallpox had scarred his eyes as a child, and to him the stars were a blur. But in 1584, Brahe had caught a guest at Uraniborg, the astronomer Nicholas Reimers Baer, copying his papers without permission. Baer later claimed many of Brahe's discoveries as his own, instilling in Brahe a deeply rooted fear of plagiarism. For this reason, Brahe gave Kepler only a few observations at a time to work on mathematically.

Within a month of starting work, Kepler threw an epic temper tantrum, what he himself described in his diary as "the rage of an uncontrollable spirit," "immoderate mental conditions," and "great insane acts," which lasted for three weeks and almost cost him his job. But Brahe, quick to forgive and hoping to make use of Kepler's mathematical abilities, agreed to his countless requests for living arrangements, free food, and time off. He even offered to secure a generous sponsorship for him from the emperor, and a nobleman's house near the imperial castle. But Brahe was adamant about one thing: Kepler would not get his hands on the forty years of observations.

On April 5, 1600, in a meeting with his employer, Kepler became enraged again and soon after sent a nasty, accusing letter filled with "unrestrained petulance" and "very arrogant sarcasm," as Brahe wrote to a friend, describing Kepler as "a rabid dog." Nevertheless, Brahe forgave him after he apologized again. In October 1601, he even introduced Kepler to the emperor and arranged for him to receive a generous income to produce new astronomical tables of planetary motions called the Rudolphine Tables.

Though Kepler and his family would be well taken care of, he must have feared he would be trapped for many years to come doing computations to boost another man's theories, never publishing his own work, never gaining the fame he dreamed of. He worried that Brahe would never publish his data or even show it to him. If Brahe died, it would go to his heirs, not Kepler. The thought that he would never get his hands on the observations drove Kepler to distraction.

A few days after Kepler's new assignment, Brahe went to his last banquet. Arriving home in agony, unable to urinate, his belly distended, Brahe fell into bed with a raging fever. For the next ten days, pain radiated throughout his body. Sometimes he was delirious, repeating over and over, "May I not have appeared to have lived in vain!" On a few occasions, after much straining, he could void a drop or two of urine. At the end of ten days, however, the illness seemed to abate. Free of pain and clearheaded, Brahe still feared he would die. He prayed and sang hymns with his family, and instructed that his observations and instruments—his most valuable possessions—go to them, not Kepler. Then he fell asleep and never woke up.

The strange death of this renowned astronomer caused many to suspect poison. The bishop of Bergen, Norway, wrote to Brahe's former assistant, "I would like to know whether you have particular knowledge about Tycho Brahe, because recently an unpleasant rumor has developed, namely that he died, but not a usual death . . . Alas, that this rumor may be wrong. God have mercy on us." The famous German astrologer Georg Rollenhagen wrote that Brahe must have been poisoned because in so "vigorous a body so drastic an effect cannot possibly result from the retention of urine."

If Brahe had been poisoned, popular opinion pinned the murder on one of two individuals. Danish King Christian IV, though hundreds of miles away, still fuming about Brahe's purported love affair with his mother, was believed to have sent Brahe's cousin Erik to give him something unhealthful to drink right before the banquet. The other suspect? None other than jealous, vicious Kepler, who had stolen the forty years of observations out of Brahe's house while the grieving family was making funeral arrangements. Kepler, instead of denying the theft, was proud of himself, boasting, "I had possession of the observations, and I refused to hand them over." Years later, he was possibly referring to the theft when he said, "Truth is the daughter of time, and I feel no shame in being her midwife."

Indeed, freed from Brahe's shadow and armed with his records, Kepler finally achieved the fame he had always desired. Shocked by the sudden loss of Brahe, Emperor Rudolph gave Kepler his position as imperial mathematician. Brahe's massive logbooks led Kepler to formulate his three laws of planetary motion, one of which is that the planets' orbits are elliptical, not circular, as had always been believed. He also developed the notion that the sun pulled the planets around by something like magnetic tendrils, a force growing stronger as the planets got closer and weaker as they moved away—breathtakingly close to the theory of gravitational attraction, which Isaac Newton would formulate in 1687 using Kepler's work.

As Kepler's fame rose, rumors that he had murdered Brahe faded. Over time, the verdict of natural illness became more common than poison. As medical knowledge improved, a popular theory speculated that Brahe died of acute uremia—the kidneys were no longer able to filter out toxins naturally occurring in his blood—probably brought on by an enlarged prostate or other obstruction of the urinary tract.

Whatever the case, Brahe's death became an important lesson for those who need to urinate.

MODERN POSTMORTEM AND DIAGNOSIS

In 1901, researchers in Prague opened up Brahe's tomb as part of their celebrations commemorating the three-hundredth anniversary of his death. They found a five-foot-six-inch skeleton in a fine silk shirt, wool stockings, silk shoes, and a hat. Though the corpse had no false nose, investigators found a crescent-shaped injury on the bridge of the nose, the exact same place where Brahe had been maimed in his youthful duel. They noticed a greenish discoloration on the area, which later tests showed was caused by brass. Either rumors of Brahe's gold and silver noses were untrue, or he donned them only for special occasions.

Though the skull had been crushed to pieces by a falling ceiling stone, a great deal of red hair remained—the eyebrows, hair on one side of the head, hair in his silk beret, and one side of a four-inch moustache. Researchers removed hairs from the moustache.

In 1991, a leading European toxicologist, Bent Kaempe, the director of the University of Copenhagen's Institute of Forensic Medicine, performed tests on the moustache hair to prove or dispel the rumors of poison. Kaempe found that in his final days Brahe suffered symptoms of severe uremia. Several things can cause this, including mercury sublimate poisoning. So Kaempe ran a test for heavy metal poisoning and found trace amounts of arsenic, which every human body has, and elevated lead levels, though not nearly enough to cause a serious illness. But the mercury level was astonishingly high, a hundred times the level of a normal modern Dane. The doctor believed Brahe's kidneys had stopped functioning as a result of a lethal dose of mercury sublimate, probably an accidental ingestion from his alchemical experiments.

But a 1996 study of the hair root showed a dramatic mercury spike thirteen hours before Brahe's death, or about nine o'clock the evening before. It appeared that Brahe may have been poisoned twice: the first poisoning on the night of the party, the second poisoning the night before he died, which killed him. Could Johannes Kepler have given him a drink with mercury sublimate before the banquet and then, ten days later when he seemed to be improving, a second dose to finish him off?

But even science is fallible. Given the sensational stories of Tycho Brahe's poisoning, a team of Danish and Czech scientists exhumed him again in 2010 and took new hair directly from his remains. Tests were conducted separately at Prague's Nuclear Physics Institute and at the Department of Physics, Chemistry and Pharmacy at the University of Southern Denmark. The new results showed that Brahe had a slight spike in mercury consumption about two months before his death, probably consumed in a medication. After that, mercury levels decreased dramatically. Analyses of samples of Brahe's bones, which would reveal heavy metal poisoning going back eight or ten years, showed that he had not consumed excessive amounts of mercury, not even in his alchemical laboratory. It was a stunning reversal of the 1990s findings that indicated murder.

So what did kill him? Most likely benign prostatic hyperplasia, known as BPH, an enlarged prostate gland. This gland surrounds the urethra, the tube through which urine flows. As the prostate grows, it can squeeze the urethra, making it difficult and even impossible to urinate. Left untreated, it can prove fatal.

Kepler is off the hook. He was a thief, to be sure, but no murderer. Though he had succeeded in attaining the fame he always wanted, his demons still haunted him. Happiness and health eluded him, and he frequently bled himself as medical treatment for his innumerable imaginary ailments or because his horoscope indicated he should. In 1630, at the age of fifty-eight, he suddenly abandoned his second wife and their young children, carting off all his possessions and leaving them penniless. While the details are vague, it seems he had fallen into a deep depression because his stars were lining up in a clear prediction of death.

A few weeks later, in the German city of Regensburg, he developed a fever, took, perhaps, too much blood from himself, and, speechless in his final delirium, kept pointing from his forehead to the heavens. The night he died, meteors streaked across the sky.

16

MICHELANGELO MERISI da CARAVAGGIO, ARTIST to ITALY'S ELITE, 1572–1610

On a hot July day in the small Tuscan seaport of Porto Ercole, a man lay dying in a hospital bed. Most likely, he could hear the sea lapping at the nearby shore and feel a cool breeze wafting in the open window, cleansing the stuffy room of the odors of sweat and bodily waste. After a lifetime of light and shadow—and very little in between—one of the world's great artists felt the darkness closing in on him, plunging him into eternal night.

Details of his death are vague, but Michelangelo Merisi, called Caravaggio after his hometown in northern Italy, was a man with many enemies, the greatest of them being himself. He had brawled, dueled, and murdered. He had been imprisoned, exiled, and pursued by bounty hunters. Had his hard living and many wounds caught up with him? Was he suffering from sunstroke or malaria? Or had one of his adversaries followed him on his journey, injuring him fatally or slipping a little something into his wine?

When Caravaggio died among strangers on his way to Rome, he was buried in an unmarked grave, as the local priest was on strike that summer. But recently, what seem to be his bones have been found, revealing important clues as to what may have contributed not only to his death but also to his extravagant, tempestuous life. For Caravaggio's powerful sense of artistic drama was eclipsed only by his boundless violence.

Though he apprenticed briefly as a teen with a mediocre artist in Milan, many art experts believe that Caravaggio was mostly self-taught. Unlike other artists of the time, he never learned to paint frescoes. He didn't produce any drawings for his pictures, nor did he draw the figures on his canvases to position them. On the contrary, he attacked the canvas in a fury, not waiting for the layers of paint to dry. He blazed his own trail through the art world, unimpeded by training.

In 1592, at the age of twenty, Caravaggio left Milan, apparently having murdered a man, and arrived in Rome, Italy's artistic capital, the dream of any painter who hoped to gain lucrative commissions from the Catholic Church. A contemporary portrait of Caravaggio shows an attractive man with thick, disheveled black hair and thick black brows, moustache, and goatee. His shapely lips are sensual. But his large brown eyes have a strange, haunted look, revealing torments of the soul.

He "goes dressed all in black," a witness in a court case said of him, "in a rather disorderly fashion, wearing black hose that is a little bit threadbare." Caravaggio's biographer, Giovanni Pietro Bellori, who was born three years after the artist died, wrote, "We cannot fail to mention his behavior and his choice of clothes, since he wore only the finest materials and princely velvets; but once he put on a suit of clothes, he changed only when it had fallen to rags."

Other than a privileged few who worked for Rome's most powerful noblemen and churchmen, most artists in Rome lived in the city's grimy underbelly in the company of prostitutes and thieves. They drank and fought and whored, competing for the same work and the same women. They insulted and attacked one another. And in between jail time, running from angry landlords demanding overdue rent, and recuperating from head-splitting hangovers and wounds incurred in brawls, some of them created magnificent art.

Much of Caravaggio's life remains as hidden in the shadows as the figures in his paintings. But Roman court records shed some light. He was involved in numerous assaults late at night, beating his victims over the head with the flat of his sword or wounding them. On April 24,

1604, he smashed a plate of artichokes into the face of a waiter whom he felt had been rude to him. He threw stones at police officers and told them to stick his sword up their arses. On more than one occasion he was arrested for defacing doors, a common insult of the time that involved throwing animal bladders of blood and excrement and painting giant erect phalluses.

In late July 1605, two women accused him of defacing their houses, and a man accused him of assault. When his landlady threw him out of her house for nonpayment of rent, he threw stones at her windows, breaking them all. Then he whacked a man on the back of his head one night in the Piazza Navona in a disagreement over a woman.

It is possible that Caravaggio was a part-time pimp. Most artists used prostitutes as models—Caravaggio certainly did—as decent women of any class wouldn't pose for them. If he were, indeed, a pimp, the strange pieces of his puzzling life make more sense. A top-rate swordsman, he would provide the women with a powerful protector, in return getting cash, respect, art models, and free sex.

Caravaggio's desires were not limited to women, however, and today we might describe him as omnisexual. Many of his contemporaries accused him of having a sexual relationship with his young assistant. His biographer and artistic rival, Giovanni Baglione, even painted an altarpiece portraying Caravaggio as Satan sodomizing Cupid.

Caravaggio apparently never spent more than a day or two in jail for his offenses as he had a powerful protector, Cardinal Francesco Maria Bourbon del Monte, a great art collector fascinated by the artist's revolutionary style. The cardinal gave Caravaggio a place to live, food, clothing, and introductions to Rome's great Church patronage system. And, with a single word, he could spring him from jail.

Caravaggio's work was compelling, disturbing, and controversial, shattering centuries of artistic tradition. No one before him had ever possessed his mastery of light and shadow—pools of light illuminating a face, a leg, a hand, spurts of blood. Nor had anyone portrayed Mary and Joseph, the disciples, apostles, and saints as real people with broken fingers, torn tunics, grimy feet, and sunburn. The real miracle, he seemed to be saying, was that God's grace could touch anyone, even those with torn tunics and dirty toenails. But Caravaggio's realism wasn't limited to human figures: his fruit was battered, the apples had worm holes, and the grapes were withered. Death and decay were everywhere around us, redeemed only by flashes of divine light.

Caravaggio's altarpieces for Roman churches astonished and amazed. No one had ever before created paintings of such drama and gritty reality. People traveled from all over Italy to see them. But while his art transfixed many, it disturbed others who saw impiety in dirty feet. Art, they believed, should not show life's warts and filth, but majestic scenes boasting a dignified cleanliness. Caravaggio's biographer Bellori wrote, "Now began the imitation of common and vulgar things, seeking out filth and deformity, as some popular artists do assiduously . . . The costumes they paint consist of stockings, breeches, and big caps, and in their figures they pay attention only to wrinkles, defects of the skin and exterior, depicting knotted fingers and limbs, disfigured by disease."

In 1605, Caravaggio painted *The Madonna of Loreto*, in which two pilgrims, a barefoot man and a wrinkled old woman, kneel before an elegant Virgin standing in a dark doorway, holding a toddler Jesus. Divine grace, Caravaggio shows us, is not reserved for the rich and powerful, but falls equally on the poor and humble. Throngs of working-class people came from near and far to see the painting. Caravaggio's enemy Baglione nearly burst with jealousy. "In the first chapel on the left in the church of Sant'Agostino," he wrote waspishly, "he painted the Madonna of Loreto from life with two pilgrims; one of them has muddy feet and the other wears a soiled and torn cap; and because of the pettiness in the details of a grand painting the public made a great fuss over it."

Caravaggio suffered some humiliating rejections because of his realism. His *Saint Matthew and the Angel* was immediately rejected due to the saint's coarse, bare legs ending in fat, ungainly feet seemingly pushed into the viewer's face. In 1606, Caravaggio delivered two more paintings that were rejected, one of them his most prestigious job yet—an altarpiece for St. Peter's Basilica.

The humiliation may have sent him over the edge. On May 28, 1606, he killed a man, a bravado like himself named Ranuccio da Terni, in a duel. No one knows why. Was it because of a prostitute? A gambling debt? An insult in the street? Wounded, knowing he would be condemned to death, Caravaggio made his way to an old family friend, the influential Marchesa Costanza Colonna. She spirited him out of Rome to her estate in the Kingdom of Naples, where he was besieged with commissions.

Even in Naples, Caravaggio must have felt unsafe—from Roman bounty hunters as well as relatives of the man he killed—because in June 1607 he left for Malta. With the aid of his princely Roman patrons, he applied to become a Knight of Malta, a military order reporting only to the pope, which offered blanket legal absolution for any crimes committed before joining. Though he didn't have the cash to buy his way into the order, he did have the talent, painting portraits of the leaders and a stunning altarpiece. After a year's trial, he became a knight, enjoying all the prestige and protection he had dreamed of. And then he seriously wounded another knight in a brawl.

Caravaggio was thrown into the *guva*, an infamous black pit carved out of the castle rock and sealed by a trapdoor eleven feet above. Somehow, after a month in the hole, he escaped, lowering himself down a sheer two-hundred-foot cliff to the sea. A couple of weeks later, he turned up in Syracuse, Sicily, some sixty miles away. Now he was hunted not only by Roman bounty hunters and Ranuccio's family, but also by the very order he had worked so hard to join. In Sicily, he continued to receive commissions. But by September 1609, he was back in Naples, apparently waiting for word from his Roman benefactors of a papal pardon. He was done with exile and longed to return to Rome.

One night in October, Caravaggio visited the Osteria del Cerriglio, a Neapolitan tavern in a narrow alleyway popular with men seeking male prostitutes. As he left the building, a group of armed men set upon him, held him down, and mutilated his face, a typical vendetta attack. Were they avenging his assault on the knight in Malta? The murder in Rome? Or something else? Caravaggio had injured and offended so many people, it is hard to say.

For six months, Caravaggio recuperated from unspecified grievous injuries at the Neapolitan villa of his patroness, Costanza Colonna. Then, in the second week of July 1610, he set sail from the Colonna Palace on a little ship called a felucca, headed for Rome with three paintings. Perhaps these were payment to a powerful cardinal for obtaining his papal pardon. It is likely that he had a traveling companion in the felucca, as the captains usually waited for at least two customers before setting out.

After a few days at sea, the felucca docked at Palo, a Spanish fort about twenty miles west of Rome. A mercantile center specializing in the transfer of heavy goods from ships to wagons and vice versa, it would have offered the artist a reliable means of transporting his three enormous crated paintings to the capital. But Caravaggio seems to have insulted a soldier checking his papers or cargo and ended up in the slammer. When he gained his freedom two days later, the felucca— with his precious paintings, his price to return home—had left.

Desperate, Caravaggio raced to Porto Ercole, which was evidently the destination of the other passenger, hoping to catch up with the ship. He must have rented a horse to ride the fifty miles. When he arrived at his destination, he collapsed. Baglione wrote with more than a hint of gleeful malice, "Finally, he reached a village on the shore and was put to bed with a malignant fever. He was completely abandoned and within a few days he died miserably, indeed, just as he had lived."

Was it heat exhaustion that killed him, riding madly along the coast in the blazing Italian summer sun, perhaps without a hat? Was it malaria, the bane of Italy? Had his lifetime of excess, including his many wounds, weakened his constitution? After all his sexual excesses, did he have syphilis? It seems, given the malignant fever, he wasn't set upon by enemies with knives, nor was he poisoned.

Or was he?

MODERN POSTMORTEM AND DIAGNOSIS

In 2010, Italian researcher Silvano Vinceti learned of a document found in the archives of the parish of San Sebastiano in Porto Ercole, written by a friar who stated the artist had died at the local infirmary and been buried in the San Sebastiano cemetery. In 1956, the burials had been cleared away to make room for new buildings and the bones placed in a bone depository at the municipal cemetery. For nearly a year, Vinceti's team examined bones, skulls, and teeth, hoping to find those that matched the artist's gender, age, build, and year of death.

Finally, tests showed that one set of bones belonged to a tall man who was between thirty-eight and forty when he died around 1610 and suffered from syphilis. Though this isn't proof of identity, it is certainly possible, especially when the bones revealed off-the-chart levels of lead.

Renaissance painters used a white paint made of lead. All that gleaming bright light in Caravaggio's paintings was made of lead white mixed with orpiment (yellow arsenic sulfide). Many artists sucked on their brushes to create a more pointed tip. He may also have absorbed the toxins through his hands by smudging his painted canvases with his fingers or paint-spattered rags and not washing afterward. No one ever accused Caravaggio of tidiness.

Arsenic and mercury, too, were abundantly used in paint. Red paint was made from realgar (red arsenic sulfide) or vermilion (mercury sulfide). It is quite possible that the temperamental Michelangelo, who died in 1564, suffered from chronic poisoning from his paints, though not enough to hasten his death; he lived to be almost ninety. Poisoning may also have affected Francisco Goya, who died in 1828; he painted directly with his fingers and absorbed the toxins through his skin. Though he lived to be eighty-two, Goya suffered a bizarre litany of physical ailments including headaches, hearing loss, dizziness, and depression. Vincent van Gogh's hallucinations and mental deterioration may have been caused at least in part by his poisonous paints.

In addition, Caravaggio probably ingested lead in his wine. Cheap wine, the kind he would have drunk in his favorite lowlife taverns, was often sweetened with lead acetate made from grapes boiled in lead containers, kept in lead pitchers, and served in lead mugs. Perhaps it's no coincidence the men who drank in such taverns were the most violent in Rome. Lead poisoning causes mood disorders, high blood pressure, difficulty concentrating, headaches, abdominal pain, and joint pain. Chronic lead intoxication from wine seems to have killed Pope Clement II in 1047 at the age of forty-two. In 1959, German researchers exhumed him from Bamberg Cathedral and found the bones of this wine-loving pontiff saturated with a fatal amount of lead.

We know that lead poisoning didn't kill Caravaggio outright because it would not have caused his fever. But it may have killed him indirectly by causing his violent encounter at the port that got him thrown in jail. And it could have compromised his general health, making him more susceptible to other ailments, such as sunstroke or malaria, tipping the artistic genius over the edge as he rode furiously along the beach.

Though Caravaggio had no known children, the team compared DNA extracted from the bones with that of people who shared his last name—Merisi—in the artist's hometown of Caravaggio. Tests revealed a genetic match of 50 to 60 percent, enough for the research team to announce an 85 percent probability that the bones were Caravaggio's. Critics of the research, however, accuse the sleepy town of Porto Ercole of staging the results to bring in tourists.

Whether Caravaggio has been found is, perhaps, not so important. What is important is whether the artist—sick, wounded, and completely abandoned, his flame guttering out among strangers—felt in his last moments the light of God's grace he had so often painted in his masterpieces.

17

HENRY STUART, PRINCE of WALES, 1594–1612

Usually the eighteen-year-old prince sprang out of bed at dawn to go hunting, play tennis, or run next to the River Thames. But in early October 1612, Henry, Prince of Wales, son and heir of King James I of England, began to suffer headaches. He had little urge to do anything other than sleep, from which he was frequently and rudely rousted by blasting bouts of diarrhea. As if the diarrhea weren't enough, his doctors believed he needed laxatives to remove the evil humors in his brain that were causing the headaches. On October 12, they opened his bowels twenty-five times with clysters—potions of turpentine and other ingredients injected into the rectum—which yielded, according to his doctor, "a very great quantity of bile, decomposed and disgusting, and at the last some phlegm."

Exhausted as he must have been from the medications even more than the illness, Henry was tasked with organizing festivities—masques, balls, and tournaments—to welcome the German prince betrothed to his sister, sixteen-year-old Princess Elizabeth, and refused to rest. Had he barred the door to the doctors and taken to bed with a bowl of chicken soup, he may have recovered quickly.

Blond and handsome, Henry embodied the hope and promise of the new Stuart dynasty, which had only come to power in England in 1603, after the death of their cousin, Queen Elizabeth. The prince excelled in all physical pursuits—hunting, riding, wrestling, tennis, swimming, tilting with lances, shooting, archery, and running—and loved everything related to warfare—military maneuvers and theory, weapons, and tournaments. When the Virgin Queen died after a long reign, there had been no royal children since the death of King Edward VI fifty years earlier, and the English people adored their young prince.

Though Henry was a talented athlete, he was a mediocre student, unlike his scholarly father or James's erudite predecessors, Elizabeth I and Edward VI. But Henry still wanted his court to be a center for study and research. To that end, he collected paintings, sculptures, and books. And while he found reading boring and, indeed, could barely sit still with a book, he was eager to learn about exploration, mining, manufacturing, and ship design. He wanted to make things, to do things. He was a future monarch in motion.

Henry doted on Sir Walter Raleigh, the explorer and scholar, whom James had imprisoned in the Tower of London back in 1603 for plotting against him. Raleigh was given comfortable apartments, however, where he read, wrote, and cooked up potions in his alchemical laboratory. Henry visited him often, asking his advice on statesmanship, navigation, and other topics. The prince was frequently heard to say that no king but his father would keep such a bird in a cage.

By 1612, James's reputation was somewhat tarnished from nine years of wild spending, love affairs with other men, and a disturbing habit of fiddling with his codpiece. He set the moral tone at his court, earning it the nickname of Sodom. English people still blushed with shame remembering the 1607 visit of King Christian IV of Denmark, the brother of Henry's mother, Queen Anne. The fourteen-day drunken orgy culminated in a feast at which the Danish monarch was smeared in jelly and cream, passed out on the floor, and was carried senseless to his royal bedchamber.

"The ladies abandon their sobriety; and are seen to roll about in intoxication," wrote Sir John Harington, Elizabeth I's godson. "I ne'er did see such a lack of good order, discretion, and sobriety, as I now have done . . . We are going on . . . by wild riot, excess, and devastation of time and temperance . . . I wish I was at home." When Queen Anne announced she would stage "a masque of maids"—a group of young virgins singing and dancing—courtiers speculated as to whether she could find any.

In contrast to Sodom, Henry's court was frugal and respectable. He even kept a swear box, where his gentlemen had to put money every time they used a foul word or took the Lord's name in vain. Proceeds went to the poor.

A stickler for duty, now, despite his illness, the prince refused to stay in bed when there was work to be done. Henry wanted to dazzle the courtiers, his sister's betrothed, and Princess Elizabeth herself with the celebrations.

On October 14, the sixteen-year-old Frederick, Prince-Elector of the Palatinate, a German kingdom, arrived for the wedding. The bridal couple had never met but were well pleased with each other, and the groom "did delight in nothing but her company and conversation," according to a contemporary report. Henry had taken an immediate liking to his future brother-in-law and spent a great deal of time with him. On October 24, the two played a tennis match at court. But by that evening, the prince could no longer power through his illness and took to his bed with a fever and violent headache.

Henry's physicians asked the king for help, and James sent his favorite doctor, Théodore de Mayerne, a thirty-nine-year-old Swiss citizen who had been physician to King Henri IV of France. Prince Frederick's team of German physicians jumped in to help, too. Naturally, with so many cooks in a kitchen, the resulting soup was very salty indeed, and the doctors spent a great deal of time arguing among themselves. Courtiers were already talking of poison and pointing the finger at the French doctor who might be working in the interests of his native country or perhaps for powerful factions in England. To protect himself, Mayerne decided to write detailed reports on the prince's illness, reports that help us understand four hundred years later exactly what happened.

Mayerne explained that Henry's natural humors were extremely warm, which he made worse by his intemperate love for exercise. "The prince continually fatigued his body by exercises and violent occupations," the physician explained, "hunting in the heat of the day, riding and playing tennis, and in consequence he often heated his blood extraordinarily (for it was his habit, having started in the morning, not to sit down all day long)." Clearly, exercise was dangerous. But so were fruit and fish, which were thought to send putrefactive humors directly to the brain. "And further," Mayerne continued, "he ate strangely to excess of fruit, and especially of melons and half-ripe grapes, and often eating his full of fish and of raw and cooked oysters beyond rule or measure at each meal, three or four days of the week."

But his riskiest behavior by far was swimming, as water opened the pores to admit evil vapors. Mayerne lamented, "He would moreover finish, in order to cool the burning heat which worked in his body during the summer, by plunging into the river after supper, his stomach full, and would remain several hours in the water. After all these irregularities, he fell ill at Richmond on the 10th of October 1612."

The morning after the tennis match, still feeling unwell but unwilling to stint God, Henry attended church twice, once in his own London palace, St. James, and later in the morning at his father's nearby palace of Whitehall. Then he dined with his father, according to Sir Charles Cornwallis in his 1626 book about the prince: "His Highness in outward appearance eating with a reasonable good stomach, yet looking exceeding ill and pale, with hollow ghastly dead eyes perceived of a great many." After dinner, the prince started to shake, sweat, and complain of a headache. He returned to St. James where, "being laid he found himself very ill, remaining all this evening in an agony, having a great drought [thirst], which after this could never be quenched but with death; his eyes also being so dim that they were not able to endure the light of a candle. This night he rested ill."

The following day the prince felt better, got dressed, and played cards with his twelve-year-old brother Charles and Prince Frederick, though he "looked ill and pale, spoke hollow, and somewhat strangely, with dead sunk eyes, his dryness of mouth and great thirst continuing. This night resting quietly." On Thursday, October 29, he rose from bed to dress but almost passed out and returned to bed. Over the following days, his fever increased and he became delirious, calling for his rapier and clothing, "crying out that he must be gone, he would not stay."

Nothing seemed to help the prince. The headaches, dizziness, drenching sweat, and buzzing in his ears increased. His breathing was shallow, his pulse rapid. His throat and tongue sprouted lesions, and his lips turned black. On November 3, he began having convulsions, his tongue was dry and furred, his thirst unquenchable, and his face was either ghastly pale or bright red. The doctors saw the prince's headaches as evidence of putrid vapors in his brain. Accordingly, they shaved his head and applied hot glass cups to the scalp, thereby drawing the nastiness into large welts. Then they split roosters and pigeons in half and applied the still-warm, bloody carcasses to his head, which they hoped would extract the noxious humors altogether. They repeatedly caused him to vomit.

Other physicians thought it best to drain the rot downward, either in the form of diarrhea or by sticking his feet between the two halves of still-warm, just-killed pigeons. In case the vapors were stuck in his veins, they bled him eight ounces at a time.

By this point, in addition to the original devastating illness, the heir to the throne was bald, dehydrated, alarmingly weak, and incontinent, voiding his waste on his sheets. His numerous doctors continued to argue with one another on a treatment plan.

King James, aware of the tumult in his son's sickroom, offered to dismiss the other physicians and leave sole charge of Henry's medical care to Mayerne. It was a sensible move, having one doctor supervising the sickroom instead of a dozen. And Mayerne possessed a sterling resume. Still, though James's offer was a great honor, it turned Mayerne's blood to ice. Prince Henry was arguably the most important person in the kingdom. If the prince died with Mayerne as the sole attending physician, he and he alone would be blamed—at best for incompetence, at worst for murder, considering he was a foreigner. Mayerne turned down the offer because, he told his friends, "it should never bee said in after Ages, that he had killed the king's elder Sonne." Those who heard this statement misinterpreted it, believing that someone else was killing the king's son with poison.

Cornwallis wrote of the prince, "The following day, Friday, November 6, . . . fainting and swooning, he seemed twice or thrice to be quite gone; at which time there arose wonderful great shouting, weeping, and crying in the chamber, Court, and adjoining streets." His "respiration became shorter, the pulse more frequent, the face redder, the tongue blacker, and the thirst greater, the tremblings [convulsions] continued, and the sighing began; in short, everything made it obvious that the blood and the humors were thrown with abundance and violence toward the brain."

In his comfortable suite of rooms in the Tower, Sir Walter Raleigh saw any possibility of his release dying with the prince. He cooked up a julep composed of compound of pearl, ammonia, musk, and bezoar stone to revive the prince. The concoction would certainly cure him, he boasted, except in the case of poison. Henry's doctors, knowing the end was coming, decided it couldn't hurt to see if the julep helped. Considering Raleigh was a traitor in the Tower, this was one case where they tested a prince's medications. It was harmless, but neither did it help.

The Archbishop of Canterbury exhorted the dying prince to trust in Jesus Christ and prepare to meet Him. By now Henry was beyond speech, so the archbishop asked him to lift up his hands as a sign of his faith and hope in the resurrection. The prince did so. From then on there was nothing more for anyone to do but wait and pray. According to Cornwallis, "His Highness, at last, half a quarter, or thereabouts before eight o'clock at night, yielded up his spirit unto his immortal Maker, Savior and Restorer, being attended unto Heaven with as many prayers, tears and strong cries as ever soul was."

The prince's mother, Queen Anne, was so heartbroken that her doctors feared for her life. Five months later, the Venetian ambassador reported, "She cannot bear to hear it mentioned; nor does she ever recall it without tears and sighs." Hearing the news of her brother's demise, Princess Elizabeth went without food for two days and cried ceaselessly. The English people were inconsolable. Cornwallis wrote, "There was to bee seene an innumerable multitude of all sorts of ages and degrees of men, women and children . . . all mourning, which they expressed by severall sorts of lamentation and sorrow, some weeping, crying, howling, wringing of their hands, others halfe dead, sounding, sighing inwardly, others holding up their hands, passionately bewayling so great a losse, with Rivers, nay with an Ocean of teares." The Venetian ambassador wrote, "So well grown was this noble tree that it promised most savoury fruit to delight the world . . . But now all these hopes are dashed by this immature and furtive demise. He faced sickness and death with the highest courage, and made his end in piety."

Naturally, rumors of poison flew across Europe. Cornwallis wrote,

"It was generally feared he had met with ill measure [foul play] and there wanted not suspicion of poison . . . Vaine rumors also have beene spread abroad, that he was poisoned." Queen Anne believed her son had been poisoned, especially since Sir Walter Raleigh said his julep of crushed pearl would otherwise cure Henry. The prince's brother, Charles, believed to the end of his life that Henry had been poisoned. Public opinion, too, came up with various reasons for the prince's murder. The Venetian ambassador to Savoy wrote, "The French ambassador said that in France they held that the Prince of Wales died of poison, and what is worse is that some hold that his father was an accomplice in the murder, as he was grown jealous of the Prince's vast designs."

Clearly the king was, at times, frustrated by his son's popularity. In 1610, when Henry's new court at St. James Palace quickly became far more sought after than his own, the king fumed, "Will he bury me alive?" But now the new heir to the throne was sickly Prince Charles, who could hardly walk on sticklike legs, probably deformed by rickets, and had a speech impediment. James murdering Henry would have put the entire Stuart dynasty at risk—something like shooting himself in the foot to spite the nose on his face. Moreover, Henry's death broke his father's heart. Months later, the Venetian ambassador reported, "The King is doing all he can to forget this grief, but it is not sufficient; for many a time it will come over him suddenly and even in the midst of the most important discussions he will burst out with 'Henry is dead, Henry is dead.'"

The king bestowed tens of thousands of pounds on his lover, Robert Carr, in distributing his son's estate. This gave rise to the rumor that Carr had poisoned the prince to obtain an inheritance. Many others insisted that staunch supporters of the Anglican Church had killed him, fearful that once he became king he would make Puritanism the official state religion. Some courtiers believed that Sir Walter Raleigh's enemies—and there were many—had killed the prince, as Henry had promised that he would have him released in December 1612, a month after he died.

The English were always ready to suspect Catholics, and French Catholics knew Henry dreamed of leading an army of Huguenots in France now that Henri IV, assassinated two years earlier, could no longer protect them. As for the Spanish Catholics, the Venetian resident in

Florence wrote, "The friends of Spain are glad at the death of the Prince. They say the remaining one [Charles] is weak and may not live long." If Charles died, the ambassador continued, "the King of Spain may one day find the way to place his foot in that Kingdom and reintroduce the true faith."

These speculations of poisoning ignored the fact that many people in London were sick and dying of a similar illness, although it was not obviously infectious. Doctors knew it wasn't smallpox, measles, plague, or dysentery, but weren't sure what it was.

CONTEMPORARY POSTMORTEM

Hoping to understand better what killed the prince and, more important, knowing that public opinion would blame someone for the poisoning (probably the French guy), Théodore de Mayerne performed an autopsy the day after Henry's death in full view of numerous physicians, surgeons, knights, and courtiers. He sawed off the skullcap and pulled out the brain, then opened the chest and stomach and removed the heart, lungs, intestines, stomach, spleen, liver, and gall bladder, passing them around for those assembled to inspect for evidence of poison or illness.

"After the opening of the most illustrious Prince," the autopsy report stated,

> we observed these things: That his liver was more pale than it
> would be, and in divers places wan, and like lead; and the gall-
> bladder was without gall and choler, and full of wind. His spleen
> was in divers places unnaturally black. His stomach was without
> any manner of fault or imperfection. His midriff was in many
> places blackish. His lungs were black, and in many places spotted,
> and full of much corruption. He had the veins of the hinder part of
> his head too full of blood, and the passages and hollow places
> of his brain full of much clear water. The truth of this relation we
> make good by the subscription of our names, November 7, 1612.

The stomach "without any manner of fault or imperfection" alone ruled out poison. The state of his other organs indicated a long and severe illness and the beginning of decomposition. The medical profession of the early seventeenth century had to leave it at that.

MODERN DIAGNOSIS

The prince's body is sealed below Westminster Abbey, unlikely ever to be exhumed (see page 110). But in 1881, a British doctor, Norman Moore, reviewed the notes on the prince's death and diagnosed typhoid fever, caused by *Salmonella typhi*, bacteria found in water and food contaminated by sewage. In Henry's time, all the bodily wastes of Londoners poured into the Thames. A generation before Henry's death, Elizabeth I, while gliding along in her royal barge from one palace to another, was so offended by the fecal odors of the Thames that she instructed her servants to burn perfume oil to protect the royal nose.

Henry probably infected himself either by eating raw oysters or swimming in the cesspool of the Thames. (Ironically, his doctors were right to warn him against both, though they were wrong about the reason.) Typhoid fever started off slowly, with headache and a slight fever, and the worst thing a victim could do was to ignore it and go about his business. The fever progressed, the patient became delirious, suffered from unquenchable thirst and migraines, and, if his natural immune system didn't overcome the infection, took about a month to die. Henry lasted twenty-seven days.

It is interesting to imagine the kind of king Henry would have been, had he lived, and safe to say that England's civil war, caused in great part by the ineptitude of his younger brother, King Charles I, would not have split the country in two. However, it is also likely that Henry, with his martial spirit, would have involved England in European wars. Dying when he did, Henry escaped having to confront the realities of seventeenth-century politics. He passed on to the realm of memory and myth unsullied, a matchless hero who never tarnished his reputation by making the wrong choices. Henry, Prince of Wales, is forever frozen in time: a golden prince, young, virtuous, and full of promise.

18

SIR THOMAS OVERBURY, ROYAL ADVISER at the COURT of JAMES I, 1581–1613

Of all the suspected cases of poisoning at royal courts, only a few have been confirmed by modern scientific analysis. But even those cases leave us with questions. Who gave Cangrande della Scala digitalis? Who killed Agnes Sorel with mercury? How did Ferdinando de Medici slip arsenic into his brother and sister-in-law's medication—if, in fact, he even did?

There is one case for which we have the answers. Let us examine the intriguing story of an unlikely murderer, twenty-two-year-old Frances Howard, Countess of Somerset, rich and beautiful, and a confessed poisoner at the court of King James I. It had all started on January 5, 1606, when her father, Thomas Howard, Earl of Suffolk, made her marry Robert, Earl of Essex, the son of Elizabeth I's swashbuckling admirer whom she executed for treason in 1601.

The marriage was doomed to remain unconsummated. At first, this was part of the plan, given the couple's youth; both were only fifteen. Though a girl could legally consummate a marriage at twelve and a boy at fourteen, many people felt that sex at such a young age could stunt growth and cause mental retardation, even death. Adolescents, it was believed, required the bodily humors voided by sex to develop their still-growing brains and other organs. They were right about early marriage endangering girls, though for the wrong reasons. An immature reproductive tract can lead to miscarriage, stillbirth, and health complications. In the developing world today, girls under twenty are twice as likely to die during pregnancy or childbirth, and girls under fifteen are five times more likely.

The Earl of Essex took off on a European tour. When he returned in 1609, nineteen-year-old Frances, who had grown into "a beauty of the greatest magnitude in that horizon," according to a courtier, found her husband a complete dolt, without humor, intelligence, or pleasant conversation. Essex, for his part, found himself completely unable to consummate the marriage. He and Frances argued about who was at fault and began to loathe each other. After a year, they stopped trying to have sex. At her annulment hearing in 1613, Frances's lawyers stated, "Desirous to be made a mother . . . she again and again yielded herself to his power, and as much as lay in her [power], offered herself and her body to be known, and earnestly desired conjunction and copulation." Despite this, Essex was "not able to penetrate into her womb, nor enjoy her."

Soon after Frances gave up hope of conjunction, copulation, and penetration in 1610, she began a flirtation—perhaps even an affair—with the sixteen-year-old heir to the throne, the subject of our last chapter, Henry, Prince of Wales, who was four years her junior. George Abbott, the Archbishop of Canterbury, wrote, "The Prince of Wales, now in his Puberty, sent many loving Glances, as Ambassadors of his good Respects."

But in the tangled web of galloping beds at the Jacobean court, Frances was also conducting an affair with the lover of Henry's father, Robert Carr, Viscount Rochester, which the prince discovered. Henry "slighted her accordingly," wrote the archbishop. "For dancing one time among the Ladies, and her Glove falling down, it was taken up, and presented to him, by one that thought he did him acceptable Service; but the Prince refus'd to receive it, saying publickly, He would not have it, it is stretcht by another."

Frances was, by this time, well stretched indeed. She had fallen obsessively, violently in love with Carr, and the fact that he was having an affair with the king only made him more attractive. King James, though he had dutifully married a Danish princess and managed to father five children, had always been strongly attracted to his own sex or, as one courtier put it, "It is thought this king is too much carried by young men that lie in his chamber and are his minions."

In 1612, James made Carr a privy counselor and put him in charge of reading foreign dispatches, summing them up, and advising the king on how to deal with them. But Carr, whose looks were of a far greater magnitude than his intellect, knew the task was beyond him and asked his other lover, thirty-one-year-old Sir Thomas Overbury, to help him. Good-looking and well educated, Overbury had a sharp mind, though his startling arrogance made him few friends and many enemies. His obnoxious personality prevented him from rising at court, but he secretly insinuated himself into the highest level of foreign affairs by helping Carr.

Overbury wasn't concerned that his lover was having an affair with the married Frances Howard. He even played the role of Cyrano de Bergerac, writing love letters for Carr. But Overbury became apoplectic in the spring of 1613 when he learned that Frances's powerful family was suing her impotent husband for an annulment due to nonconsummation, and Carr actually intended to marry her. Overbury called Frances a whore, a slut, and other vile names to Carr and anyone else who would listen. Carr's servants reported hearing loud arguments between the two men.

Essex, displeased to be called "my lord gelding" as he walked the halls of Whitehall Palace, contested the annulment, asserting that he felt he could have sex with a woman one day, just not with the most beautiful woman in England right now. The stern bishops set to hear the case debated whether they should put asunder what God hath joined together if sex was even theoretically possible. But they certainly would not grant the annulment if they knew for a fact that Frances had been sleeping around.

Frances began to obsess that Sir Thomas Overbury's increasingly shrill vilification of her reputation would imperil her annulment and her subsequent marriage to the love of her life. It would be so much easier if her annoying husband died; that way no annulment would be required. According to later court records, Frances gave a fortune-teller a diamond ring to procure a poison which "would lie in a man's body three or four days" before taking effect, "and that this poison was . . . to be given to the Earl of Essex." Sadly for Frances, the fortune-teller ran off with the ring.

Frances and Carr needed to get Overbury out of the picture, one way or the other. It seems Carr suggested that King James appoint him England's new ambassador to Russia, and the king—who never liked Overbury and wanted him as far away as possible—eagerly agreed. Surprisingly, Overbury refused the appointment outright. Perhaps it was the freezing, barbarous destination, or maybe he wanted to stay near Carr to prevent his marriage. It is also possible that Carr advised him to refuse, knowing the king, furious at being disobeyed, would throw Overbury into the Tower. Which is exactly what happened on April 21, 1613.

Overbury was out of the way just in time. On May 15, the annulment commission opened its hearing on Lady Frances's marriage, an embarrassing four-month-long investigation into erections, nocturnal emissions, and the tedious complexities of church law. Some on the commission had heard of Frances's scandalous reputation and insisted that she be examined by a panel of women to make sure she was a virgin. Her aghast family, claiming such an examination would outrage the girl's modesty, insisted she wear a heavy veil during the examination, a stratagem they used to substitute another girl in place of Frances. The court roared with laughter when the commission found that she was both "fit for carnal copulation and still a virgin."

As the commission ground forward, the Howard family, not content with throwing Overbury in the Tower, wanted to make sure he never regained his liberty to slander them again. Frances's great-uncle, the powerful Earl of Northampton, arranged to replace the Lieutenant of the Tower, a respectable fellow named Sir William Wade, with Sir Gervase Elwes, a gambler deeply in debt who would do the bidding of the Howards. At Frances's instigation, Northampton hired a man named Richard Weston to attend Overbury. Frances's friend and coconspirator, Anne Turner, sent Weston a phial "full of a water of a yellowish and greenish color," according to his later testimony, which he was told to give Overbury and make sure that he himself didn't drink. Assuming that Elwes was in on the plan, Weston, preparing to give Overbury his supper, asked him, "Sir, shall I give it to him now?" When Elwes asked what he meant, Weston produced the poison and explained that the countess had told him to mix it with Overbury's food.

Horrified, Elwes harangued Weston on eternal damnation and made him pour the brew down the drain. Weston thanked him for saving his soul. Convinced he wouldn't try to poison Overbury again, Elwes didn't fire Weston, nor did he tell anybody about the attempt on Overbury's life. Surely no one would believe that the powerful Howard family would resort to poisoning a prisoner.

Anne Turner then consulted with Dr. James Franklin, a hunchbacked, shady character whose face was ravaged by syphilis. She wanted a poison that wouldn't kill its victim quickly, but would "lie in his body for a certain time, whereby he might languish away by little and little." Dr. Franklin sold her a liquid that she tried out on a cat, which began "wailing and mewing as it would have grieved any to have heard her," and died two days later. Finding the poison too strong—surely it would raise suspicions—she asked for others. Dr. Franklin later testified that he brought her seven kinds of poison including mercury water, cantharides, and white arsenic.

Soon Frances was baking poisoned tarts and jellies in her kitchen and sending them to Overbury, though pretending that they had come from Carr, who assured his old friend in numerous letters that he was trying to get him released. Frances instructed Weston "to give Sir Thomas the tarts and jelly, but taste not thou of them." Sir Elwes, who claimed he didn't know the food was poisoned, stored them in the Tower kitchens. Within a short space of time, he found the tarts had turned "black and foul" while the jellies had grown a kind of fur. He told Frances's delivery boy that Overbury didn't want any more, and by July they stopped coming.

During his trial, Dr. Franklin told of efforts to make Overbury's poisoning look like a languishing illness, with just enough poison given at each meal to make him sick. "There were continual poisons given him in all his meats," Dr. Franklin testified, "and that Overbury being once desirous to eat of a pig, they provided him a pig, and in the sauce they put white arsenic. Sir Thomas Overbury did eat neither broth nor sauce for the most part but that there was poison put into it, so prepared to lie in his body before it wrought." He continued, "Sir Thomas Overbury never ate salt but it was poisoned with white arsenic, and that the salt was provided by Mrs. Turner and prepared by her in her chamber. And once, Sir Thomas Overbury being desirous to eat of a partridge, and the sauce being water and onions, cantharides, being black, was strewed therein instead of pepper."

By early July, Overbury was having bouts of fever, not a symptom of heavy metal poisoning. But he had many symptoms that were: nausea, vomiting, and diarrhea. He suffered unbearable thirst, weight loss, and "loathing of meat." His urine had a pungent odor and his skin became so sensitive it tortured him to wear clothes.

It is possible that, in addition to the poison Frances was sending him and the natural illness that caused his fever, Overbury was simultaneously being killed by his well-meaning doctors. His murder investigation looked into his prescription medications and found that one apothecary required twenty-eight sheaves of paper to list them all. The apothecary testified he saw medicine in Overbury's chamber that he had not prescribed, including potable gold. Overbury must have had the constitution of an ox to survive as long as he did—almost five months.

The physician who treated Overbury most often was Théodore de Mayerne, the court doctor who had treated Prince Henry a year earlier in his last illness. Mayerne routinely prescribed mercury for a variety of ailments. Furthermore, he believed an effective means of voiding bad humors was to open a vein and keep it open by inserting seven peas into the wound. Then he slapped a plaster on top of it, a process that could cause gangrene to set in.

One of Mayerne's favorite recipes was called balsam of bats, which called for boiling "three of the greater sort of serpents or snakes cut into pieces, two very fat sucking puppies, one pound of earthworms washed in white wine; common oil; malago sack [a sweet, white Spanish wine], sage, marjoram, and bay leaves." Two pounds of hogs' lard were stirred in. When the puppies and snakes started to disintegrate and decompose, the fat was removed and "the marrow of a stag, an ox's legs, liquid amber, butter and nutmegs" were mixed in. Mayerne also believed in frequent enemas to void nasty humors downward.

Carr sent Overbury a special medication to use in an enema, a powder that, according to Dr. Franklin, was "white arsenic and was sent to him in a letter. The poison being heavy worked upwards and downwards." Its effects were disastrous. Instead of acting as a gentle laxative, it provoked some sixty fits of diarrhea and vomiting in a few hours.

Yet when Overbury's servant reported this to Carr at Whitehall Palace, Carr asked how sick his master really was. "Yea, my Lord, in great danger of death, for he hath had threescore purges and vomits in one day." Carr cried "Pish!," smiled broadly, and sauntered away.

The only thing that kept poor Overbury going was the belief that his friend and lover, Robert Carr, was assiduously working at court to get him out of prison. Then Overbury received a letter from his brother-in-law—probably smuggled in, as his mail was restricted—disabusing him of this notion. Carr was, in fact, responsible for his long imprisonment. Overbury flew into a fury and wrote Carr a letter threatening to let everyone know of his affair with Frances. The annulment suit was grinding toward its conclusion—with judges seeming to be evenly split—and Carr and Frances could not afford Overbury ruining everything by blabbing about their adultery.

According to Sir Elwes's testimony, Frances bribed the apothecary's boy to fill a syringe with sulfuric acid instead of the herbs usually used in enemas. The doctor, unaware of the poisonous contents, gave Overbury the enema on the evening of September 14. Almost immediately Overbury was in agonizing pain, his shrieks and groans so loud they penetrated the thick Tower walls. The following morning he was dead, and the apothecary's boy had disappeared.

The body, which was described as having "looked like poison itself," started decomposing immediately, and the stench was unbearable. No one wanted to poke around the foul corpse. The coroner, having heard of the deceased's ill health all summer, quickly returned a verdict of death by natural causes and fled the death chamber for some fresh air. When Overbury's parents asked for his remains, they were told that due to "the unsweetness of the body, the keeping of him above ground must needs give more offence than it can do honor."

Traditionally, corpses were wound tightly in a sheet. But Overbury's attendants, unwilling to touch the stinking corpse, threw a sheet on top of it. He died at seven o'clock in the morning; by three that afternoon he was buried beneath the altar of the Tower church, St. Peter ad Vincula, taking his place along with scandalous personalities of the

Tudor era: Anne Boleyn, George Boleyn, Catherine Howard, and Lady Jane Grey.

Frances must have heaved a huge sigh of relief when Overbury finally died. Eleven days later, she heaved another one: seven of the twelve commissioners investigating her annulment suit sided in her favor. She was no longer married to the impotent Earl of Essex. On December 26, during the court's Christmas festivities at Whitehall Palace, she married Robert Carr, whom King James had made the Earl of Somerset as a wedding present.

In August 1613, the king fell madly in love with the chestnut curls and well-turned legs of a twenty-two-year-old commoner named George Villiers. Carr had alienated many at court with his arrogance, and these enemies now championed Villiers at Carr's expense. Erupting in fury, Carr chastised James, who distanced himself from his former lover.

In the summer of 1615, King James heard rumors that Frances and Carr had poisoned Overbury in the Tower. At first the king thought it was a lie created by the pro-Villiers camp to smear Carr. But then Carr stupidly demanded the king issue a blanket pardon for whatever crimes he may have committed in the past. Suspicious now, the king refused and ordered a full-scale investigation into Overbury's death. Over the ensuing months, Anne Turner, James Weston, Sir Richard Elwes, and Dr. James Franklin were found guilty of murder and hanged. Robert Carr was imprisoned in the Tower. Frances, heavily pregnant, was confined to her Whitehall Palace apartments.

On December 9, Frances gave birth to a girl. As she recovered, James sent her word that only if she confessed and asked for pardon would he consider showing her mercy. On January 2, she made a full confession of Overbury's murder, stressing that her husband was entirely innocent. The Spanish ambassador reported, "She spoke to them plainly, confessing the part which she had taken in desiring and aiding the death of Overbury, as being a girl aggrieved and offended by the most unworthy things which he had said about her person, but that the earl of Somerset—who at that time was not yet her husband—neither knew anything about it nor took any part in it . . . For all this she threw herself at the feet of the king, begging for his grace and pity."

On January 19, the Somersets were formally indicted as "accessories to murder before the fact done." On April 4, 1616, Frances moved to the Tower. When she learned that she was in the same room where Overbury had died, she became so hysterical they moved her. Her trial opened on May 24. Frances, dressed elegantly in black, wept copious, shimmering tears as she pled guilty and begged the court for mercy. The court sentenced her to death—that she should "be hanged by the neck till she were stark dead," though everyone in the courtroom knew she was too noble, too female, and far too beautiful for that to happen. It must have been particularly galling for her to see among the spectators the smirking face of her former husband, the Earl of Essex.

Carr was less amenable to persuasion than his wife. He continued insisting he never knew anything about the plot to poison Overbury, and all the other witnesses who said so were lying. He admitted sending his friend the white enema powder, but maintained he had thought the medication would help him.

Carr admitted that he had not tried to dissuade the king from imprisoning Overbury, "to the end that he should make no impediment in my marriage." However, he denied that he had convinced his friend to refuse the Russian posting and insisted he had told him to take it. He also admitted that he had sent Overbury tarts in prison, but wholesome ones. Any poisoned tarts must have come from Frances.

Like Frances, Carr was found guilty and sentenced to hang, though James had no intention of hanging him any more than he did Frances. But neither could he set them scot-free. The king feared a public outcry against the injustice of pardoning nobles while hanging lesser folk guilty of the same crime. He stripped Carr of his titles and properties and kept him and Frances in the Tower—living in the same apartment—until 1622. James pardoned Carr in 1624 and returned some of his forfeited property.

After everything they had done to be together, Frances and Carr found no happiness in their marriage. Neither one could ever return to court, and Carr seemed angrier at her for ruining his career than for murdering his friend. His replacement in the king's bed, George Villiers, continued to rise, becoming the Duke of Buckingham, while Carr sat stewing in the country with a wife he resented. According to one courtier, Frances, who continued to love him, was "dead whilst living, being drowned in despair."

Frances died in unbearable pain at forty-two, according to her autopsy report, killed by "a disease in those parts below the girdle," a sure sign of God's punishment. Her uterus was "cancerous in the whole body of it." And a tumor in her right breast "had penetrated and wrapped itself about the ribs on the inside."

Frances never became pregnant after the birth of her daughter in 1615, possibly because of a gynecological problem resulting from the delivery. Her daughter, Anne Carr, grew up to be one of the great beauties of the court of Charles I. In 1637, she married William Russell, the future Duke of Bedford, for love, a marriage her father secured by promising a dowry he didn't have. Consequently, relations between Robert Carr and Anne soured, and when Royalist troops ransacked his house in the early 1640s, he accused his daughter of organizing the raid to steal his tapestries. Carr died at the age of fifty-eight in 1645, the middle of the English civil war, a curious, scandalous relic from a bygone era.

Interestingly, during Carr's trial, the attorney general, Sir Frances Bacon, gave voice to one aspect of the case that outraged all good Englishmen: that they should be tarnished with cowardly crimes usually committed by sinister Italians. Poisoning, Bacon declaimed, was "a foreign manslayer fetched from Rome . . . an Italian revenger, a stranger to the records of England."

The fear that the English, as much as the Italians, would bear the stigma of poisoners came true for a time. Sir John Throckmorton, England's ambassador to the Netherlands, wrote that Overbury's poisoning had sullied England's reputation abroad. "They begin to brand and mark us with that hideous and foul title of poisoning one another," he wrote, "and ask if we become Italians, Spaniards or of what other vile, murderous nation."

19

PRINCESS HENRIETTA STUART of ENGLAND, DUCHESSE d'ORLÉANS, 1644–1670

On June 29, 1670, Princess Henrietta Stuart, the duchesse d'Orléans, drank a glass of chicory water prepared by her lady-in-waiting. Almost immediately, Henrietta grabbed her side and gasped out that she had been poisoned. Nine hours later, after suffering unendurable agonies, she would be dead at the age of twenty-six.

The daughter of Charles I of England and Henrietta Maria of France, Henrietta had grown up at the French court during the English civil war—in which her father lost his head—and the Protectorate of Oliver Cromwell. Though unfashionably thin, Henrietta was a pretty girl with blue eyes and chestnut hair. "She dances with incomparable grace," wrote a contemporary, "she sings like an angel, and the spinet is never so well played as by her fair hands."

The princess was almost universally beloved for her sweetness. Another courtier wrote, "That which the Princess of England possessed in the highest degree was the gift to please, and what we call grace; these charms were diffused over all her person, over all her actions, and her mind, and never was princess so equally capable of making herself loved by the men and adored by the women." She had the charm of her maternal grandfather, French king Henri IV, it was said, and of her paternal great-grandmother, Mary, Queen of Scots.

In 1660, her older brother, Charles, was invited to return to England as king, and Henrietta, no longer a poor exile, was suddenly a shining star on the royal marriage market. Soon a husband was found for her in her cousin, the younger brother of King Louis XIV, Philippe, duc d'Orléans. Known throughout Europe as Monsieur, the prospective bridegroom "was well-made and handsome," according to a courtier, "but with a stature and type of beauty more fitting to a princess than a prince. And he had taken more pains to have his beauty admired of all the world than to employ it for the conquest of women . . . His vanity it seemed, made him incapable of affection, save for himself." He also liked to wear women's clothing.

The chronicler of Louis's reign, the duc de Saint Simon, described him later in life: "Monsieur was a little round-bellied man, who wore such high-heeled shoes that he seemed always mounted upon stilts; was always decked out like a woman, covered everywhere with rings, bracelets, jewels; with a long black wig, powdered, and curled in front; with ribbons wherever he could put them; steeped in perfumes, and a fine model of cleanliness. He was accused of putting on an imperceptible touch of rouge."

When he was seventeen, Monsieur had been "corrupted" in the "Italian vice" by the handsome nephew of the queen mother's lover, Cardinal Jules Mazarin, and had taken several male lovers since then. But at the age of twenty, Monsieur decided he was in love with Henrietta and wanted nothing more than to marry her. Seeing his extravagant infatuation with her, many at court hoped the lovely princess would cure him of his homosexual inclinations.

Henrietta, while not in love with him, genuinely liked him. They had grown up together, and he could be hilariously funny. They married in March 1661, when Henrietta became officially known at the French court as Madame. But, as Henrietta's good friend, Marie-Madeleine Pioche de La Vergne, comtesse de La Fayette, wrote, "The miracle of inflaming the heart of this prince was not given to any woman upon earth." His passion for her ebbed within months of the wedding, and he fell madly in love with Philippe, chevalier de Lorraine, a love that would continue until Monsieur's dying day decades later. The chevalier was "as beautiful as an angel," all agreed, as well as "insinuating, brutal and devoid of scruple."

Though Monsieur was clearly bisexual, he fathered eight children with Henrietta (only two girls survived), and three with his second wife. In the 1670s, his second wife reported that he wore clanking rosaries and saints' medals on his private parts during sex in the hopes that they would enable him to be fruitful and multiply, and it is possible he did this with Henrietta, as well.

Monsieur soon became jealous of his wife's popularity. People generally liked her better than they did him, and he couldn't bear it. Even his own brother, King Louis, became infatuated with her. Growing up, Louis had found Henrietta skinny and unappealing. Yet as soon as she married Monsieur, he saw her in a new light—as a desirable woman. The romantic attachment was so obvious that many at court believed that Monsieur's first child was, in fact, his niece. More galling to Monsieur than the love affair between his brother and his wife was the fact that Henrietta was receiving more attention and respect from the king than he was. His soaring passion for her had faded to indifference soon after marriage, but now it degenerated into sputtering, seething resentment.

Soon the king's wandering eye fell upon Henrietta's lady-in-waiting, the sweet, pretty Louise de La Vallière, whom he made his mistress. Madame, perhaps to avenge herself on the king, began having an affair with one of her husband's lovers, the extravagantly bisexual Armand de Gramont, comte de Guiche. There was "great acrimony on every side," according to a contemporary report. The comte de Guiche argued bitterly with Monsieur, who was both his lover and the husband of his lover. Then Monsieur fell in love with François de la Rochefoucauld, Prince de Marsillac, but he, too, was in love with Madame, which made Monsieur despise his wife even more.

For the next several years, Henrietta's life was a tangle of love affairs, stolen letters, treacherous servants, secret assignations, lovers hiding in chimneys from her husband, and vicious intrigues, the actors wearing exquisite costumes and playing ridiculous roles on gorgeous sets. In short, it was a kind of real-life *opera buffa* except no one was singing.

Monsieur gave Henrietta's spending money to the chevalier de Lorraine, forcing her to pawn her jewelry to pay her servants. Then he installed the chevalier in the finest rooms of his palaces and allowed him to run the household; the chevalier insolently issued orders to Henrietta herself.

By the winter of 1669, Henrietta's life had become so miserable that she complained to both King Louis and King Charles about the disgraceful treatment meted out to her by the chevalier de Lorraine. In January 1670, Louis finally imprisoned the chevalier before exiling him to Rome with a huge annual pension for services rendered to his brother. Monsieur was devastated and blamed Henrietta for sending away the love of his life. The heat of his fury congealed to cold suspicion when he frequently found Louis and Henrietta closeted together, their conversation ending awkwardly when he clattered in. According to a courtier, "Monsieur was extremely vexed to see his wife—with whom he was already displeased—suddenly acquire such importance in the eyes of the King, and although he guessed she must be involved in some affair of consequence he was quite unable to find out what it was."

Louis knew that his brother was a gossiping chatterbox who told his male lovers every thought in his head. He certainly couldn't be trusted with state secrets. And Louis was working with Henrietta on a secret treaty between France and England that she would personally take to her brother, Charles II, to sign. Bursting with jealousy, Monsieur refused to let her go to England, then insisted that he accompany her, to no avail. Finally, sullenly, he relented.

In May 1670, as their carriage bounced over the road to the coast where Henrietta would board ship, Monsieur cast her a coldly appraising glance. An astrologer, he said, had predicted he would have more than one wife. Referring to her bouts of ill health, he added waspishly, "Evidently Madame will not live long, so the prediction seems likely to be fulfilled."

Beginning in 1667, Henrietta had had "a pricking in her side," according to her dear friend, the comtesse de La Fayette, "which forced her to ly downe 3 or 4 houres together on the ground finding no ease in any posture she placed herself in." By April 1670, her condition worsened. When she suffered these attacks, she subsisted mostly on milk, the only thing that didn't upset her stomach.

But Henrietta sparkled with health and gaiety on May 25, when she and her entourage of two hundred courtiers and servants docked in Dover. She was as delighted to see her beloved brother again as she was to be away from her objectionable husband. "Madame is in perfect health," wrote Charles Colbert, marquis de Croisy, the French ambassador to England. Over the next two weeks, she spent many hours in meetings—the treaty was ratified June 1—but she also attended court dinners and balls and sailed with her brother in yachts along the coast. These were the happiest days of her life and were over all too soon.

On June 16, Henrietta returned to Paris. Due to the stifling heat, on June 24 the court left for the more refreshing air of the château of Saint-Cloud, just three miles west of Paris on the Seine. The king's cousin, Mademoiselle de Montpensier, wrote, "She went to the queen's room like a dressed-up corpse with rouge on its cheeks and when she went out, everybody including the queen, said that she had death written on her face."

A few days later, feeling another stomachache coming on, Henrietta invited the comtesse de La Fayette to join her at Saint-Cloud. It is fortunate for us that she did. The comtesse penned an extraordinary blow-by-blow account of Henrietta's death. "I arrived at Saint-Cloud on the Saturday, at ten o'clock at night," she wrote. "I found her in the garden; she said that I would not find her looking well, for in truth she did not feel it." Henrietta's stomach pains soon abated, and the following afternoon, "Madame de Gamaches [a lady-in-waiting] brought to her, as well as to me, a glass of chicory-water that she had asked for some time previously." (Chicory is a leafy plant much like endive and used in salads; its roots are used to make a coffee substitute, which is probably what Henrietta drank.) The comtesse de La Fayette continued:

Madame de Gourdon, her lady of the bedchamber, presented it. She drank it, and replacing with one hand the cup upon the saucer, with the other she pressed her side, and said in tones which betrayed great suffering: 'Ah! What a pain in my side! What agony! I cannot bear it.' She flushed as she uttered the words, and a moment later her color faded to a livid pallor that alarmed us all. Her cries continued, and she bade us take her away, as she could no longer stand. . . . We supported her by the arms. She walked with difficulty, bent almost double. She was undressed in a moment. I held her up while they unlaced her. She was still complaining of the pain, and I noticed that there were tears in her eyes.

Once in bed, Henrietta "began to cry out more loudly than before, flinging herself from one side to the other, like a person in fearful agony." Monsieur was summoned, as was her doctor, who diagnosed her ailment as gas. The comtesse continued,

> Madame still cried that she had fearful pains in the pit of her stomach. All at once she bade us look to the water she had drunk, saying that it was poison; that perhaps one bottle had been mistaken for another; that she was poisoned, she knew it well, and that she would be given an antidote.

Standing next to Monsieur, the comtesse observed him carefully:

> He seemed neither embarrassed nor upset at Madame's thought. He said that some of the water must be given to a dog; he concurred in Madame's opinion that oil and counter-poison should be sought, to banish from Madame's mind so distressing an idea. Madame Desbordes, her chief waiting-woman and her most faithful servant, answered that she had mixed the water herself, and had drunk of it.

A dog was rounded up in the palace—we can only imagine the panic of its owner—and given the chicory water, which it lapped up cheerfully as everyone studied it. Nothing happened. Perhaps it wagged its tail.

Monsieur's valet brought Henrietta a traditional poison antidote, powder of vipers, and the doctors gave her other remedies that made her vomit and soil her sheets. "The trouble of taking all these remedies," the comtesse reported, "and the excruciating pain she suffered, brought her to a prostration that we took for relief, but she said that her sufferings were just as great, that she had no longer the strength to cry out, and that there was no cure for her complaint."

Royal physicians who galloped in from Versailles and Paris agreed she was merely suffering from gas. "We stayed talking round the bed, believing her to be in no danger," the comtesse de La Fayette wrote. "We were almost consoled for the pains she had suffered, hoping that the condition she had been in would serve to bring about her reconciliation with Monsieur; he seemed to be touched." But when Henrietta heard someone saying she was getting better, she replied, "All that is so far from the truth that were I not a Christian I would kill myself, so fearful are my pains."

When physicians held candles up to examine her face—which was beginning to look like that of a corpse—Monsieur asked if it annoyed her. "Ah, no, Monsieur," she answered, "nothing can annoy me anymore. Tomorrow morning you will see, I shall no longer be alive."

Madame de La Fayette continued:

She was given some soup, for she had taken nothing since dinner. As soon as she had swallowed it, her pains redoubled, becoming as violent as they had been after the glass of chicory water. Death was clearly seen in her face, and she endured the most terrible sufferings without the least sign of fear. When the King [Louis XIV] arrived, Madame was in the paroxysm of agony . . . The king, seeing that so far as one could tell there was no hope for her, wept and bade her good-bye. She spoke to him, begging him not to cry, for his tears affected her deeply, and adding that the first news he would hear on the morrow would be that of her death.

When Lord Montague, the English ambassador, arrived, Henrietta:

spoke of the king, her brother, and of the grief her death would cause him . . . She begged the Ambassador to send him word that he was losing the person who loved him most in all the world. Then the Ambassador asked her if she had been poisoned. I know not if she answered that she had been, but I do know that she told him to say nothing about it to the King, her brother, that at all costs he must be saved this pain, and particularly that he must not think of vengeance. She said that the King [Louis XIV] was not guilty, and that no blame must be laid at this door . . .

Meanwhile, she was growing weaker, and every now and then a faintness came upon her, which affected her heart. Doctors wanted to bleed her by opening a vein in her foot and placing the foot in hot water. "If you wish to do it," she said, "there is no time to be lost; for my head is growing confused and my stomach is filling." Her physicians tried to bleed her, but no blood came. She thought she would die while her foot was in the water. "The priest gave her a crucifix, she took it and kissed it ardently. Her strength failed her and she let it fall, losing the power of speech at almost the same moment as her life. Her agony lasted but a minute and after one or two little convulsive movements of her mouth, she expired at half-past two in the morning, nine hours after she had been taken ill."

All fingers pointed immediately at Monsieur. When Charles II heard of the death of his twenty-six-year-old sister, whom he had seen radiantly healthy just days before, he exclaimed, "Monsieur is a villain!" Her admirer, the Duke of Buckingham, insisted that England declare war on France for murdering an English princess. People rioted in the streets of London, crying "Down with the French!" Charles sent guards to protect the French embassy against violent mobs.

CONTEMPORARY POSTMORTEM

Louis, too, suspected that someone—either his brother or the chevalier de Lorraine from afar—had poisoned Henrietta. He arranged for an autopsy the day after her death, witnessed by seventeen French and two English doctors; the English ambassador, Lord Montague; and about a hundred others, including many Englishmen. The marquis de Saint-Maurice attended the autopsy and wrote, "The stomach of the princess had swollen in the most extraordinary way since her death. The very first incision into her body released such a vile stench that all those taking part in the dissection were obliged to withdraw, and could only approach the corpse once more after furnishing themselves with masks against this evil odor . . . The body was found to contain a great quantity of bile, and the liver was quite putrid."

Her stomach—which would have shown damage if poison had been involved—looked healthy, except for a "a hole with blackened lips." When the English surgeon Alexander Boscher wanted to inspect the hole more closely, the French physician in charge told him it was nothing, just an incision he had inadvertently made with his autopsy scissors.

The physicians concluded that an imbalance of overheated bile had caused Henrietta to die from cholera morbus—an inflamed intestinal

tract that has nothing to do with the bacterial infection called cholera
that first appeared in Europe in the nineteenth century.

MODERN DIAGNOSIS

Henrietta's body was destroyed in the wholesale plundering of the
royal vaults of Saint-Denis in 1793. But history has proved that Alexander Boscher had been on to something. Doctors at the time knew that
corrosive poisons could indeed perforate the stomach, and the French
physicians, fearing war with England, must have seen with horror the
black hole in Henrietta's stomach. But they didn't know that a poison-
induced perforation would be large and circular with dark ragged
edges, while hers was small with round black lips—what we know today
as the sign of a perforated gastric ulcer.

Henrietta had had the symptoms of an ulcer—periodic stomachaches,
heartburn, and nausea—for three years. On June 29, 1670, as she sipped
some chicory water, the ulcer burst, allowing stomach acids to flow
into her body cavity. She felt the sharp stab of the rupture, which she
thought was poison. She then suffered unbearable pain as the acid
inflamed her other organs, causing nausea, vomiting, diarrhea, and
death—symptoms similar to arsenic poisoning. The soup she ate in her
sickbed leaked out of her stomach into her abdominal cavity, causing
her yet more agony.

Tragically, Henrietta's daughter with Monsieur, Marie Louise, queen
of Spain, suffered similar symptoms immediately before her death, also
at the age of twenty-six, in 1689. For years, Marie Louise had eaten
mostly oysters, olives, and cucumbers, just as her mother had only
consumed milk for weeks at a time, possibly because these foods did
not irritate a gastric ulcer. At five o'clock on the morning of February 10, 1689, Marie Louise awoke with excruciating pain, vomiting,
and diarrhea, and died two days later. Marie Louise had so feared being
poisoned at the treacherous Spanish court she had asked Louis XIV for
antidotes. Everyone at the courts of both France and Spain believed she
had been murdered for not giving her impotent husband, the horrifi-
cally inbred Carlos II, an heir. But in retrospect, it is possible she inherited
from her mother a genetic predisposition to gastric ulcers.

If the European medical community had widely published and dis-
seminated case studies as they do now, the doctors at Henrietta's

autopsy may have understood what really killed her. Only five years earlier, in 1665, a renowned twenty-seven-year-old portrait painter in Bologna named Elisabetta Sirani died within twenty-four agonizing hours of suffering sudden and severe abdominal pain. The city's top surgeon performed the autopsy in front of seven physicians and discovered a hole in the stomach, ringed by hardened tissue, which he believed was caused by corrosive poison.

Elisabetta's distraught father convinced local authorities to charge her maidservant with murder. At the trial, two doctors testified that Elisabetta had died of poison, while two others believed that the hole in the stomach was caused by an ulcer. The maid was given the benefit of the doubt and found not guilty. We can only wonder how many innocent servants were, in fact, executed for poisoning because their employers died of ruptured ulcers.

As for Monsieur, after he dutifully married Elizabeth Charlotte, Princess Palatine—the no-nonsense German wife Louis had picked out for him—the king permitted the chevalier de Lorraine to return to court. The new Madame told her many friends she believed Henrietta had indeed been poisoned, but that Monsieur had had no knowledge of it. He was such a gossiping tattler he would have bragged about killing her at some point, she knew, but instead he just seemed mystified by her death.

Elizabeth Charlotte tried to keep on relatively good terms with the chevalier de Lorraine and Monsieur's many other male lovers, even though they stole her money, cosmetics, gowns, and jewelry. She feared they might offer her some chicory water, too.

20

MADEMOISELLE de FONTANGES, MISTRESS of LOUIS XIV of FRANCE, 1661–1681, and the AFFAIR of the POISONS

As the exquisitely beautiful mistress of King Louis XIV lay dying in a Paris convent, she told anyone who would listen that someone was slowly poisoning her. Wracked with constant pain, coughing and bleeding vaginally, Marie-Angélique de Scorailles, duchesse de Fontanges, had no idea that confessed poisoners sitting in a nearby jail had already corroborated her story.

The daughter of the noble but impoverished comte de Rousille, Marie-Angélique had been graced with such astonishing good looks that her relatives, "having more love for their fortune than for their honor," according to the court wit Roger de Rabutin, comte de Bussy, "clubbed together to fit her out for Court, and to provide her with means corresponding to the position she was entering." In other words, they hoped Louis XIV would choose her as his mistress. In October 1678, they obtained for her the highly visible position of lady-in-waiting to Madame Palatine, the second wife of the king's brother, Monsieur, whose first wife was Henrietta, the subject of our last chapter. In her new position at court, Marie-Angélique became known as Mademoiselle de Fontanges for a property her family owned.

The king had had several mistresses by then, each one well rewarded for her services. His first mistress, the gentle Louise de La Vallière, had lasted from 1661 to 1667, when she was pushed aside by the witty, ravishing Athénaïs, marquise de Montespan. The marquise became the star of the world's most glittering court. Her Versailles apartments consisted of twenty rooms, while the queen had only eleven. Dripping in jewels, she reveled in the king's love and the power it gave her.

But Louis's eye wandered so often that she could never relax. One after the other, women tumbled cheerfully into the king's bed, hoping to oust Madame de Montespan as official mistress, but somehow she managed to retain her position. In 1678, after she gave birth to her ninth child (two with her husband and then seven with the king), she did not regain her figure. On one occasion when the Italian writer Primi Visconti saw Madame de Montespan getting out of her carriage, he was shocked at how fat she had become. Having caught a glimpse of her thigh, he crowed that it was the same size as his waist.

And then Mademoiselle de Fontanges landed on the scene. The girl's looks caused courtiers to burst into fits of poetry. One ambassador wrote, "An extraordinary blonde beauty, the like of which has not been seen at Versailles in many a year. A form, a daring, an air to astonish and charm even that gallant and sophisticated Court." The king was immediately smitten when he saw the girl in his sister-in-law's fragrant retinue of lovely ladies and made her his mistress by early 1679. Madame de Montespan pretended to find solace in religion—fasting, praying, and meeting with her confessors. Many a cast-off royal mistress did the same, "bestowing the dregs of her beauty on Jesus Christ," as the English wit, Sir Horace Walpole, put it. But the tempestuous marquise couldn't always keep up this display of admirably piety. Sometimes she broke down in tears and, oblivious to the irony, decried "the great sin committed by Mademoiselle de Fontanges." Courtiers were treated to the sound of the king and his longtime mistress berating each other, their angry voices echoing down gilded palace halls.

While Madame de Montespan's vanity, pride, and temper had made her few friends at court, everyone acknowledged her great wit and amusing conversation. Those who spoke to Mademoiselle de Fontanges, however, were deeply disappointed the moment she opened her mouth. One courtier called the new mistress "beautiful as an angel and stupid as a basket." A resident noblewoman at court, Marthe-Marguerite de Caylus, wrote, "The King, in truth, was attracted solely by her face.

He was actually embarrassed by her foolish chatter . . . One grows accustomed to beauty, but not to stupidity."

Though the king realized the girl was stupid, he just couldn't deny himself her beauty. On New Year's Day 1680, Mademoiselle de Fontanges appeared "looking like a goddess" and shining in jewels at a celebratory mass attended by the king. Louis started wearing coats that matched her gowns, which they both trimmed with identical ribbons.

Courtiers were surprised when, on January 16, Mademoiselle de Fontanges failed to appear at the wedding of Mademoiselle de Blois, the king's thirteen-year-old daughter with Louise de La Vallière, to the prince de Conti. They soon discovered that the king's mistress had had a miscarriage. But miscarriages, stillbirths, and the death of infants happened often enough, and everyone assumed she would return to her radiant self quite quickly.

On February 27, she appeared at a ball, as lovely as ever. But courtiers noticed a new fragility about her and remarked that she barely danced at all. On April 6, the king gave her the status of the duchesse de Fontanges, endowing her with a staggering annual pension of 80,000 livres. Madame de Montespan writhed with fury. Despite all their years together and all their children, the king never made her a duchess because that would make her unpalatable, estranged husband a duke. Yet this stupid chit of a girl, without wit or education, who hadn't given the king even one child, obtained the honor Madame de Montespan had longed for all her life.

As a duchess, Mademoiselle de Fontanges even received the much-coveted tabouret, a tasseled wooden folding stool upon which the lucky few derrieres could sit in the presence of the royal family. It was carried pompously about by a bewigged and liveried servant, who snapped it open with a flourish and set it down when the duchess was ready to be seated. The marquis de la Fare reported, "Madame de Montespan was close to bursting with spite, and like another Medea, threatened to tear their children limb from limb before the very eyes of the King."

Despite Madame de Montespan's rage at the girl's duchy, some courtiers observed that the honor "smells of dismissal" and might be a retirement present, exactly the kind he had given Louise de La Vallière right before he chucked her out of his bed to make room for Madame de Montespan. "Wit is necessary to make love last," wrote the comte de Bussy, "and Fontanges is very young to have it." He was being generous. Aging does not usually render a stupid person a genius. All Mademoiselle de Fontanges offered was her sex appeal, and that had dwindled due to the lingering complications of her miscarriage. She was suffering from "a very stubborn and disobliging loss of blood," according to a courtier, that rendered sex unappealing. After a time, her face became puffy and her entire body swelled a bit. Since she could offer the king neither sex nor enjoyable conversation, she had become useless to a man who required his women to have at least one or the other, and preferably both. One courtier wrote on July 3 that the king regarded Mademoiselle de Fontanges with "extreme indifference" and that she cried often, knowing she had lost his love.

On July 17, she set off for the abbey of Chelles to visit her sister, the abbess. The celebrated letter writer Marie de Rabutin-Chantal, known as Madame de Sevigné, watched the imposing cavalcade of six coaches, each pulled by six or eight horses, and ruminated on the unimportance of wealth without the health to enjoy it. "The beauty losing all her blood," she wrote, "pale, altered, overwhelmed with sadness, thinking nothing of the forty thousand écus of income and a tabouret, which she has, and desiring health and the king's heart, which she does not."

Languishing in her sickbed, by September Mademoiselle de Fontanges began speaking of poison. What she did not know—in fact, what only a handful of people at the top levels of government knew—was that several criminals operating a poison ring confessed to a plot to kill both her and the king on behalf of none other than the vengeful rejected mistress, Madame de Montespan.

The extraordinary events that became known as the Affair of the Poisons began in 1676 when the lovely young marquise de Brinvilliers was executed for poisoning her father and two brothers. She had hinted darkly that her actions were fairly common among all levels of society—even the rich and noble. When the chief of the Paris police investigated, he found a thriving underworld of witchcraft and poison run by several hundred criminals working as fortune-tellers who would happily do anything for the right price. They read palms and tarot cards and sold love potions. Some of them took fraud to a higher level. One self-proclaimed sorcerer told a client to bury twelve gold pieces under a certain tree and, when he returned, it would have multiplied. He returned to find an empty hole in the ground and the fortune-teller vanished.

More disturbingly, the police discovered that some fortune-tellers performed abortions and conducted Black Masses where babies were sacrificed, invoking devils to do the client's bidding. They also sold poisons to rid their well-heeled customers of enemies, irritating spouses, and rich relatives who refused to die in a timely manner. On February 22, 1680, one of the chief sorceress-poisoners, known as La Voisin, was executed for witchcraft. Her twenty-two-year-old daughter, Marie Montvoisin, was kept for questioning, and it was she who revealed what her mother had only hinted at: that certain noblewomen, slavering for the wealth and power that came with being the king's mistress, tried to free up the position by poisoning those who held it.

According to Marie Montvoisin, in 1661 when, at the age of twenty-three, Louis had taken Louise de La Vallière as his mistress, at least two countesses had asked the fortune-tellers for poison to kill her so they could have a crack at getting the job. If they did manage to slip something toxic into her soup, it didn't hurt her; Louise lived in rude good health until old age. Then, in 1667, Madame de Montespan wanted the plum position. She tried a different tack; when her good friend Louise invited her to private dinners with the king, Madame de Montespan poured love potions into his wine and food—disgusting concoctions of dead baby's blood, bones, and intestines, along with parts of toads and bats—in the hopes of making him fall in love with her.

Marie Montvoisin described Black Masses performed to win the king's favor, held in abandoned chapels and officiated over by a defrocked priest named Guiborg, with the holy chalice held on Madame de Montespan's naked groin:

> At one of Madame de Montespan's Masses, I saw my mother bring in an infant, obviously premature . . . and place it in a basin over which Guiborg slit its throat, draining the blood into the chalice . . . where he consecrated the blood and the wafer . . . speaking the names of Madame de Montespan and the King . . . The entrails were taken the next day by my mother . . . for distillation, along with the blood and the consecrated Host . . . all of

which was then poured into a glass vial which Madame de Montespan came by, later, to pick up and take away.

Either because of her scintillating wit or the love potions, the king duly dropped Louise and took Madame de Montespan as his mistress. But having attained her heart's desire, she couldn't afford to relax for a moment. It seemed every woman at court was boldly offering herself to the king, and the virile monarch often accepted. Marie Montvoisin reported, "Every time something new came up to upset Madame de Montespan, every time she feared a diminution of the King's good graces, she came running to my mother for a remedy, and then my mother would call in one of the priests to celebrate a Mass and then she would send Madame de Montespan the powders which were to be used on the King."

According to the girl's testimony, when Mademoiselle de Fontanges arrived at court late in 1678 and enslaved the king, Madame de Montespan—who was twice her rival's age, bad-tempered, and grown blowsy with childbearing—decided to take matters further. She would kill both the king and her rival by poison and offered La Voisin the enormous sum of 100,000 écus to carry out the murders. "Oh! What a fine thing is a lover's spite!" La Voisin reportedly exclaimed.

Marie Montvoisin explained that an acquaintance of her mother's named Romani planned to pose as a silk merchant and offer Mademoiselle de Fontanges some gorgeous poisoned cloth, which would kill her if she wore it. If she turned down the cloth, he would offer her a fetching pair of poisoned gloves, which would prove too great a temptation for a lady to resist. They would send the victim into a slow decline, eventually killing her.

The king, however, they would kill quickly. On certain days, he allowed his subjects to give him petitions requesting any number of things—the pardon of a prisoner, the righting of an injustice, or royal intervention in a lawsuit. He often read two or three as the petitioners waited on bended knee for his decision, but most petitions were placed on a table for his later perusal. La Voisin and her coconspirators wrote a request for the release of a prisoner and then steeped the paper in a deadly poison. Upon opening the petition, the king would be overcome by fatal fumes and die on the spot.

La Voisin used her connections to arrange for a valet at the palace of Saint-Germain to make sure she would be among the first to have an audience with the king. She set out on Sunday, March 5, 1679, but returned to Paris four days later in a foul mood. She had not been able to get near enough to the king to hand him the petition directly. She could have laid it on the table but feared a royal servant would open it and die instead of the king. She announced she would return to the palace on Monday, March 13, and try again. But when a group of priests paid her a visit on Friday, March 10, she wondered if the police were planning to arrest her for witchcraft and burned the petition. On Sunday, March 12, she was indeed arrested and began spewing confessions and accusations that hinted at—but did not name—a powerful lady at court.

When, in the course of the lengthy investigation, Louis realized Madame de Montespan was involved, he panicked. There was no question of allowing the police to interrogate his mistress of thirteen years, and the mother of his children. Louis would be the laughingstock of Europe if word got out that he had ingested babies' blood and bats' wings. He shut down the entire investigation. Witnesses who had even mentioned her name were either executed or locked in solitary confinement in distant fortresses until their deaths, with their jailers under strict orders never to speak to them.

Though the king kept Madame de Montespan at court and treated her with painful respect, he always visited her with his brother in tow and never again ate or drank anything in her presence. For he finally understood why for twelve years he had awoken with a headache sometimes after having dined with her the night before. He was revolted at the quantities of noxious potions he had consumed over the years, but perhaps he was even more disgusted at the behavior of the woman he had loved.

While the investigation made clear that Madame de Montespan had ordered love potions for the king, her involvement in the plot to kill him and Mademoiselle de Fontanges is less certain. We must bear in mind that La Voisin herself was dead by the time investigators heard these tales from her daughter. Furthermore, the contingent of criminals involved in the case changed their stories frequently during the months of incarceration, pointing fingers at one another and "remembering" new information that might bring about improved prison conditions or a lighter sentence. Additionally, the purported means of poisoning is highly dubious. We now know that it would have been impossible for anyone to die from wearing a poisoned gown or gloves. Corrosive substances could have caused a skin rash, but nothing more harmful. And the fatal fumes rising from a letter are laughable—we can only wonder how the poisoners didn't end up poisoning themselves during its preparation—though no one involved in the investigation seemed to doubt that such things were possible.

It is also important to point out that by the time Mademoiselle de Fontanges became sick in January 1680, from complications of a miscarriage, the scurrilous gang of poisoners had been sitting in jail for ten months. But so widespread were the tentacles of actual murder and poison in Paris that many believed someone had, in fact, managed to get to Mademoiselle de Fontanges. They reasoned that perhaps she would have recovered from the miscarriage if someone hadn't kept poisoning her.

After an illness lasting a year and a half, Mademoiselle de Fontanges died on June 28, 1681, shortly before her twentieth birthday. When the king heard the news, he made it clear that he didn't want an autopsy, presumably because he feared the revelation that Madame de Montespan really had poisoned the girl. But the distressed family of the deceased, seeing their good fortune melting away before their very eyes, insisted.

CONTEMPORARY POSTMORTEM

The six physicians who conducted the autopsy found that Mademoiselle de Fontanges's lungs were severely diseased—the right one was full of pus—while her chest was flooded with liquid. Her liver and heart were described as "blighted," whatever that meant. There is no mention of any irregularity in the stomach, the foremost sign of poison.

MODERN DIAGNOSIS

Though Mademoiselle de Fontanges's body was destroyed during the French Revolution, later physicians, intrigued by her unusual constellation of symptoms, have tried to diagnose her fatal illness. One early twentieth-century doctor believed that she had died from pleuropneumonia induced by tuberculosis. However, in view of the fact that she is known to have suffered from a persistent loss of blood after her miscarriage, a more recent authority suggested that when she lost her baby, a fragment of the placenta lodged in her uterus. This would have been a source of infection, which ultimately brought about an abscess on the lungs. Whatever she died of, it certainly wasn't poison, despite all of Madame de Montespan's purported efforts.

The Italian writer at Versailles, Primi Visconti, concluded it was the miscarriage that killed the girl, who had died "a martyr to the king's pleasures." But most people believed that poison had done the trick and that Madame de Montespan—with her shrewish ways, raging jealousy, and aging looks—had been behind it. Courtiers took to staring at their food before they touched it, wondering. Visconti wrote, "Almost no one trusted his friends anymore . . . As soon as someone felt ill from having eaten too much, he believed he had been poisoned." Normal cases of stomach upset now resulted in urgent antidotes, self-induced vomiting and diarrhea, accusations of attempted murder, and numerous cooks thrown into jail. One wit remarked that if all the bad cooks in Paris were seized, the prisons would soon be overflowing.

21

WOLFGANG AMADEUS MOZART,
IMPERIAL COURT MUSICIAN,
1756-1791

On November 20, 1791, thirty-five-year-old Wolfgang Amadeus Mozart took to bed in his Vienna apartment with a fever. Most likely, it didn't worry him much. Since childhood he had survived countless serious illnesses: smallpox, jaundice, typhus, tonsillitis, gastric disorders, recurring strep throat, and upper respiratory infections. He had always bounced back with renewed creative energy to dazzle the world with his music.

This time, however, it would be different. After the great composer died in agony on December 5—his swollen flesh emitting a nauseating stench, his puffy face almost unrecognizable—whispers arose of poison administered by his jealous, vengeful musical rival at the Austrian imperial court, Antonio Salieri.

The soaring exultation of late eighteenth-century music gives no sign of the treachery involved in its creation. It was an era when the most talented composers scrambled desperately for the few court musical positions. The gold lace and diamond buttons, the satin knee breeches and silk coats concealed cutthroat ambition, backstabbing, dirty tricks, betrayals, and conspiracies.

Mozart had known this life since earliest childhood. His father, Leopold, served as vice *Kapellmeister*, or music director, at the court of the prince-bishop of Salzburg and taught music to both his children: Maria Anna, called Nannerl, born in 1751, and Wolfgang, born in 1756. Under his father's rigorous tutelage, Wolfgang began to play the harpsichord at the age of three. At five, he was composing his own tunes.

Starting when Wolfgang was six, Leopold spent several years with his wife and children touring the glittering courts of Europe as he monetized his two child prodigies. Nannerl played beautifully, but little Wolfgang—engaging and self-assured—astonished his audiences with his talent. He could even play blindfolded. By the time Wolfgang was nine, he could read any piece of music, improvise on any musical theme given him, and name any note he heard. He had an astounding musical memory; he could hear a piece comprising many instruments and voices, come home, and write it down. At the age of eleven, he had a hundred compositions to his credit: arias, dances, and symphonies. No other musician had ever written so much music at such an early age.

Leopold's practice regimen was harsh, and many wondered how the slight, fragile boy survived it. Not only did he study the piano, violin, and other instruments, but he also had to master foreign languages, as all court musicians did. Despite his frequent illnesses, Wolfgang's wholehearted passion for music kept him working at a frenetic pace.

Leaving his mother and sister at home, Wolfgang and his father continued to travel around Europe, with Wolfgang performing, composing, attending operas and musical events, and meeting famous composers to expand his knowledge. At each court, Leopold tested the waters for an official court position for his son. It was the surest way for a composer to receive a substantial regular salary, along with great prestige. As far as writing music was concerned, a composer received payment only for the first performance. There were no copyright laws or royalties. No positions materialized, so Wolfgang's father took him home.

Given the magnitude of the boy's talent, it seems to us unfathomable that he couldn't land a job. But there were, in fact, several reasons for this. For one thing, he did not fawn over the crowned heads of Europe and sometimes openly disdained them. He believed that everyone was equal except, of course, in terms of their talent. "It is the heart that ennobles man," he wrote. Indeed, the more he saw of royalty, the less he liked it. When, in 1781, he met Archduke Maximilian Franz, a son of Austrian empress Maria Theresa, Wolfgang wrote his father that "stupidity oozes out of his eyes." The chief chamberlain of Salzburg's prince-bishop—his father's employer—found the young composer so impudent he threw him out of the palace with a hard kick to his rear end. Second, most courts wanted Italian musicians, as they were quite in fashion, and hiring a Germanic music director instead of an Italian one was something like hiring a cook from Poland instead of France.

Moreover, Mozart's music was revolutionary, disturbing. Not for him the pleasant, feckless tunes that delighted the rich and noble, but new, difficult music that challenged the soul. Many people either didn't understand it or didn't want to make the effort. After Mozart's first performance of his opera *The Abduction from the Seraglio*, a perplexed Emperor Joseph II came up to him and harrumphed, "Very many notes, Mozart." To which the composer replied, "Exactly as many as needed, Your Majesty." Furthermore, Mozart composed mostly instrumental music. When he did compose vocal music, he shifted the emphasis away from the singers and toward the music, which disgruntled not only the audience but also the prima donnas of the opera world.

Leopold tried to stunt his son's musical expression, forcing him to write whatever was popular to earn money. Despite the father's constant complaints of debts and poverty, he lived in an eight-room apartment with attached stables and kept a fashionable carriage. He had accumulated large sums of money thanks to his son's performances for the crowned heads of Europe. One of the few people who ever saw his collection of carefully hoarded gifts—expensive snuffboxes, elegant watches, ivory canes, silver platters, and gold tableware—remarked that it was "like inspecting a church treasury."

At the age of twenty-five, Wolfgang decided it was time to get out from under his father's control and spread his wings as both an artist and a person. In March 1781, he arrived in Vienna, capital of the Austrian empire, a city that offered countless musical opportunities with some three hundred thousand inhabitants and numerous concert halls, music academies, and a talented musical community. And it was there that he finally found his home. Mozart earned money from performing at academies, at subscription concerts, and in the homes of wealthy patrons. He gave private piano lessons—though it is hard for us to imagine taking a piano lesson from Mozart—and writing music. But in the end, he worked harder to earn far less than many musicians who lacked his genius.

Mozart's chief rival in Vienna was Antonio Salieri, a successful Italian composer who wrote operas in three languages. He dominated opera in Vienna during Mozart's adult career and was appointed imperial *Kapellmeister* in 1788. Mozart wrote his father several letters complaining that Salieri and his minions blocked his every attempt to obtain an official position. For instance, in 1781, when Mozart thought the emperor would hire him to teach piano to Princess Elisabeth of Württemberg, the fiancée of the emperor's nephew, Joseph II gave the post to Salieri. "The emperor has spoilt everything," Mozart wrote bitterly, "for he cares for no one but Salieri."

Nevertheless, Mozart and Salieri seemed to have had a mutual respect for each other's musical talents. In 1785, the two composed a cantata together, and in 1788, Salieri produced Mozart's *Figaro* at court instead of one of his own operas. When Salieri saw Mozart's *The Magic Flute* for the first time in 1791, according to Mozart, "He heard and saw with all his attention, and from the overture to the last choir there was not a piece that didn't elicit a 'Bravo!' or 'Bello!' out of him."

Unlike the grave, dignified Salieri, Wolfgang was not an imposing figure. As one of his piano pupils wrote, "He was small of stature and of a rather pale complexion, his physiognomy had much that was pleasant and friendly, combined with a rather melancholy graveness; his blue eyes shone brightly." The 1984 movie *Amadeus* captured the manic side of Mozart's character, the practical jokes, dirty witticisms, and love of laughter. In 1782, he wrote a canon in B-flat major he titled *Lick My Ass Right Well and Clean*.

The Austrian novelist Karoline Pichler, a piano student of Wolfgang's, wrote a revealing anecdote. One day while they were playing a duet— she on the bass, he on the piano—"he suddenly tired of it, jumped up, and in the mad mood which so often came over him, he began to leap over tables and chairs, miaow like a cat, and turn somersaults like an unruly boy."

Ironically, the eternal child in the Mozart family wasn't Wolfgang; it was Leopold, sulking, petulant, and victimized, seething with resentment in Salzburg that his son had finally eluded his viselike grasp and was finding some success in Vienna. His frequent letters berated Wolf-gang with accusations of laziness, wastefulness, ingratitude, disobedi-ence, and incompetence. In September 1781, Mozart wrote his father resignedly, "Do trust me always, for indeed I deserve it. I have trouble and worry enough here to support myself, and it therefore does not help me in the very least to read unpleasant letters."

In 1782, at the age of twenty-six, Mozart did what Leopold had al-ways feared—he married. He had first met Constanze Weber and her musical family a few years earlier, in Mannheim, Germany, during a trip with his mother. Leopold had been furious at his son's obvious in-fatuation with the oldest of the four sisters, Aloysia, and, without ever having met them, insisted that the entire greedy family was trying to ensnare his talented son for the purpose of getting his earnings for themselves. Now, four year later, Mozart had reconnected with the family in Vienna, where they had moved, and fallen in love with the third sister.

Leopold must have been beside himself when he received Mozart's letter announcing the engagement. His son was out of his power for-ever now because of that woman. Father and son only saw each other twice more during uncomfortable visits. Leopold died in 1787 at the age of sixty. Mozart didn't go to his father in his last illness, nor did he attend the funeral.

Ironically, soon after Leopold's death, Mozart finally received the official court position his father had tried so hard to obtain for him. Emperor Joseph II hired him as a court chamber musician to write minuets. In his final years, with the composition of four successful op-eras, Mozart's income increased significantly. However, he was always behind on bills as he spent generously on clothing, fine dining, gifts for Constanze, and gambling. That fall of 1791, Mozart enjoyed good health, writing letters about the delicious food he feasted on—pork cutlets, capons, sturgeon—and composing gorgeous new music in a nonstop frenzy. Perhaps it didn't surprise those close to him that he had finally run himself down enough to get a fever.

But this illness, unlike all his others, didn't fade away. When Mozart swelled up so grotesquely he was unable to move, his wife and her sister, Sophia, made him a special gown that opened in the back to make it easier to get a chamber pot beneath him and wash him. On December 4, he became delirious. His two doctors took between two to three liters of blood from Mozart, reducing his body's ability to fight the infection. The following day, Mozart shuddered, vomited a spume of brown liquid, and fell back dead.

His widow, Constanze, privately told her friends that her husband had died of a fever. But left with two small boys, a heap of debt, and no income, she publicly fueled rumors of poison to increase sympathy for herself. She spoke of a mysterious masked stranger who commissioned a Requiem Mass. As Mozart wrote the music, the story goes, he grew seriously ill. "I know I must die," Mozart reportedly said. "Someone has given me acqua Toffana [arsenic] and has calculated the precise time of my death, for which they have ordered a Requiem, it is for myself I am writing this." But the truth was much more banal. A few months before Mozart's death, the eccentric count Franz von Walsegg hired him to write a Requiem Mass to commemorate the recent death of his wife. Secrecy was important because the count, an amateur musician, wanted to pretend he had written the music himself.

Unburdened by the facts, Constanze obtained a pension from the emperor and arranged profitable concerts of her late husband's music. It is far more interesting to listen to the music of someone who was mysteriously murdered than someone who died of a natural illness. Soon Constanze became wealthy.

Most people thought Mozart's archrival, Salieri, was responsible. In his last surviving letter, dated October 14, 1791, Mozart wrote from Prague, where the court was staying, that he picked up Salieri and the soprano Caterina Cavalieri in his carriage and drove them both to the opera. Salieri would have had the opportunity to pass Mozart a flask of alcohol in a carriage ride, for instance, or add a little something to his wine over a private dinner discussing the latest opera.

Salieri never lived down the rumor of having murdered Mozart, even though he took over the musical education of Mozart's younger son. With Salieri's instruction, Franz Xaver Wolfgang Mozart became a famous composer and conductor himself. At the end of his life, Salieri suffered from periodic bouts of dementia during which he admitted killing Mozart. But in his lucid moments he steadfastly denied doing so. In 1823, one of Ludwig van Beethoven's pupils, Ignaz Moscheles, visited the ailing seventy-three-year-old Salieri in the general hospital outside Vienna. The composer hastened to tell him, "Although this is my last illness, I can assure you on my word of honor that there is no truth in that absurd rumor; you know that I am supposed to have poisoned Mozart. But no, it's malice, pure malice, tell the world, dear Moscheles, old Salieri, who will soon die, has told you."

According to another poison theory, the Freemasons murdered Mozart because he, a Mason since 1784, had revealed many of their secrets in *The Magic Flute*. But far from reviling Mozart, his fellow Freemasons held a Lodge of Sorrows for him. The writer of *The Magic Flute*'s libretto, Emanuel Schikaneder, was also a Mason, and he lived unmolested by murderous Masons for another twenty-one years.

MODERN DIAGNOSIS

The most ridiculous part of the murder story is that many people in Vienna were dying of the same illness that killed Mozart. "Acute military fever" was listed as the cause of death on Mozart's death record. We are not sure what acute military fever was, and researchers have come up with no less than 118 possibilities. One is rheumatic fever, but this illness usually causes shortness of breath, a symptom not mentioned in contemporary reports of his illness. Besides, its victims are usually children, and when it does attack adults, they have joint pain, not swelling.

Given the swelling—the medical term is edema—and the stench, it is clear that Mozart's kidneys had stopped functioning. When the kidneys fail, waste products are not evacuated in the urine but build up in the bloodstream and are released in sweat, saliva, and other secretions until the entire body reeks of urine, a condition called uremic fetor. But not all kidney diseases would have caused Mozart's shocking edema.

One illness does explain all these symptoms. *Streptococcus equi* attacks the glomeruli, the kidneys' microscopic filters, sending waste throughout the body instead of into the urine. As its name suggests, it is primarily a disease of horses and cows. But like anthrax, it is highly contagious not just to other animals but also to humans. Mozart, dashing around in a carriage, would have been frequently exposed to horses and may have drunk unpasteurized milk.

Sadly, there is no autopsy report to help us better understand what might have killed Mozart. As far as his doctor was concerned, the cause of death was clear: the current epidemic of acute military fever. And even if family members had wanted an autopsy, the body was in such a state of swollen, reeking decay—and quite possibly infectious, to boot—even the most stoic physician would have been reluctant to cut it open. Nor are there any remains to study, as Mozart's bones are lost to history. Reeling from the egalitarianism of the French Revolution, Emperor Joseph II, in an attempt to curb vainglorious funerals, had passed laws to keep them modest. Mozart's remains, therefore, were transported at night with no funeral procession to St. Marx Cemetery outside the city walls. As a result, none of his friends or family members saw the location of the grave. In addition, Joseph's edicts required that "middle-class" coffins be interred five to a grave pit and dug up after ten years to make room for new coffins.

The sexton of St. Marx, however, one Joseph Rothmeyer, claimed he had marked the spot where the renowned composer's coffin was buried. Ten years after Mozart's death, in 1801, Rothmeyer duly dug up a skull that he proudly displayed as Mozart's; the skull now rests in the Mozart Museum in Salzburg. Unfortunately, he dug up the wrong skull. The jawless cranium bears clear evidence of a fracture, and Mozart never fractured his skull. But, in a stunning reversal of logic, some historians believed the skull proved that Mozart had actually died of a blow to the head. This theory vanished in 2006 when the Mozart Museum tested the skull's mitochondrial DNA against that taken from the thigh bones of Mozart's maternal grandmother and his niece. There was no evidence of any genetic relation.

While we will probably never know for sure what killed Wolfgang Amadeus Mozart—it's safe to say it wasn't a cracked skull—perhaps it doesn't matter in the end. The only thing that counts is that he lived and still lives in his hauntingly beautiful music. But though we are grateful for his gifts that abide with us—626 works in all, operas, symphonies, string quartets, minuets, masses, and piano concertos—we grieve at the loss of what he would have created had he lived longer than his allotted span of thirty-five years. That heartbreakingly exquisite music, captured in eternity, hovers just beyond our reach.

22

NAPOLEON BONAPARTE,
EMPEROR of FRANCE, 1769–1821

The unrelenting abdominal pain was like a knife slicing through flesh and muscle and organs, again and again, day after day, week after week, without the relief of death.

Napoleon Bonaparte had risen from nowhere to become the most powerful person on earth. He had ruled an empire of his own making that, at its apogee, stretched from the Atlantic Ocean to Russia, from the icy Baltic to the sapphire-blue Ionian Sea, and comprised some seventy million souls. Now he was emperor of two rooms in a rat-infested, mildewed house on a rock in the middle of the Atlantic Ocean. Soon, his empire would shrink even further, to a wooden box six feet long, two and a half feet wide, and two feet high.

On April 15, 1821, he wrote in his will, "I die prematurely, assassinated by the English oligarchy and its hired killer: the English nation will not be slow in avenging me." After two more weeks of agony, he added, "After my death, which cannot be far off, I want you to open my body . . . I recommend that you examine my stomach very carefully, make a precise, detailed report on it . . . I bequeath to all the ruling families the horror and shame of my last moments."

Indeed, his death would cause the crowned heads of Europe to pop the champagne corks. King Louis XVIII of France—the old, cowardly, unpopular brother of Louis XVI—sat uneasily on a sagging throne. Many Frenchmen longed for Napoleon to come back yet again with the energizing spirit of the Revolution. Britain, which had taken custody of Napoleon, feared he would escape the island, round up another army, and attack England, despite the fortune they spent annually on keeping him in exile. And the kings of Germany, Austria, Spain, Italy, and Russia would have loved to see him safely buried if, that is, his death seemed natural. News of his murder would surely cause revolutions to spring up in Napoleon's name.

The man who convulsed the Western world more than anyone since Alexander the Great was born in modest circumstances to minor nobility in Corsica, an island off the west coast of central Italy. There were eight children to feed, educate, and dower, which became quite difficult after Napoleon's father, Carlo Buonaparte, a lawyer, died from stomach cancer in 1785 at the age of thirty-eight.

Devoted to his mother and siblings, Napoleon worked hard to rise in the world to help support them financially. He graduated the École Militaire—the eighteenth-century French version of West Point—at the tender age of sixteen, using his math skills to specialize in artillery. To fit in with his French colleagues, in his twenties he changed his name to the more French-sounding Bonaparte. When the Revolution started in 1789, Napoleon was a strong supporter. He saw how little justice and equality there was for the common man in a society ruled by selfish royalty and sneering aristocrats.

Rising quickly through the ranks, in 1796 the twenty-seven-year-old was made full general and took his army to northern Italy. In just thirteen months, Napoleon scored jaw-dropping victories against forces four times the size of his own. He was bold, decisive, and courageous, completely unrattled on the battlefield as bullets whizzed around him. When the horse he was sitting on took a bullet and keeled over, he would casually step off the carcass and mount a fresh steed. "If your number is up, there's no point in worrying," he said.

Above all, it was his imagination that won him victories. He confounded his enemies by doing the unexpected, including marching all night long. His energy and endurance were almost superhuman. He could work twenty-four hours a day with a couple half-hour naps. Moreover, Napoleon inspired great loyalty among his men, many of whom he knew by name, by sharing their hardships and dangers.

Napoleon left Italy with two new republics firmly allied to France. In December 1797, he arrived in Paris a national hero. Frenchmen wanted to learn more about this new Achilles. They found the conquering general quite handsome, with his chiseled face, light brown hair, and gray-blue eyes. He was five foot six and a half inches tall, average for the time, with a lean frame. He so hummed with energy that he became easily bored and could rarely sit still. He loved to ride for hours on end and often paced while talking.

Soon, Napoleon was on his way to Egypt, which he conquered easily. He then set about exploring with the scientists and academics he brought, and building roads, hospitals, and schools.

When he returned to Paris in October 1799, he found that France possessed 167,000 francs in cash and debts of 474 million. Civil servants hadn't been paid in months. Unemployment was skyrocketing. Bandits terrorized travelers. Clearly, the disorganized French government needed a strong leader to set the nation on the right path. In a spectacular flurry of wheeling and dealing, Napoleon staged a coup and named himself First Counsel of France. He borrowed from banks and raised money from lotteries. He created a new, efficient tax department that quickly brought in income and property taxes. He spent wisely and balanced the budget. Gold coins replaced worthless paper money.

French laws were confusing and often contradictory. Napoleon, believing that the law should be clear and accessible to every citizen, developed a new system of laws known as the Napoleonic Code. Radically modern for the time, it assured the people of France equality before the law, the inviolability of property, and an end to feudal privileges.

He built roads, increased the production of crops, and nearly tripled French silk production. He unlocked the ghetto gates and invited the Jews to come out, live and work wherever they wanted, and to vote as full French citizens. He created the first professional fire brigades and introduced free vaccination and public trials by jury. Annoyed by the age-old difficulty of finding houses and businesses—addresses were quite vague—he numbered every building, inventing the system we use today with odd numbers on one side of the street and even on the other.

Napoleon made himself emperor of France in December 1804. Though he had become the most powerful man in the world, he liked to speak of his humble Corsican origins and called the throne "a piece of wood covered in velvet." Many guests at his coronation were astounded to see the newly minted emperor yawning during the hours-long ceremony.

As emperor, Napoleon's economic and administrative progress was extraordinary. Soon, France enjoyed full employment and stable prices. People paid their taxes. Crime was drastically reduced. Children went to school. In short, under Napoleon France quickly became more prosperous than it had been in well over a century. As he conquered more territory—Spain, Germany, Holland, Belgium, Switzerland, the rest of Italy, Poland, Dalmatia—he exported the benefits of justice, prosperity, and governmental efficiency. Naturally, however, many of the conquered bristled under a new regime—no matter how enlightened—forcibly put in place by a French nobody.

In 1810, Napoleon divorced his wife, Josephine, the seductive Creole he had married in 1796, because she had given him no children. Two months later, he married the pretty but stupid daughter of Emperor Francis II of Austria, Marie Louise, who soon presented him with a son.

Though he made alliances with Austria, Russia, Sweden, and Denmark, the constant thorn in his side was Great Britain, which did not want peace. The British government blushed with shame at the thought of Yorktown—their humiliating loss to that other group of ragtag revolutionaries, the Americans—in 1781, and considered a peace with Napoleon as another slap in the royal face. To the British, seeing this nullity crown himself emperor was nothing short of sacrilege. They were further horrified when, as kingdoms toppled, Napoleon replaced the scions of inbred, mildewed royal dynasties with his own parvenu brothers and sisters. The British convinced Napoleon's allies to break their treaties and become his enemies.

The turning point for Napoleon was the ill-fated invasion of Russia in 1812. Estimates vary, but the emperor went in with between 450,000 and 600,000 men from across the empire, and came out with between 40,000 to 70,000. The following year, a coalition of Austria, Sweden, Russia, Great Britain, Spain, and Portugal formed to fight him and beat him back with their superior numbers. By the time Napoleon returned to Paris, the city had surrendered to the enemy, and his wife and son had been taken to Austria by his father-in-law, Emperor Francis II. Napoleon abdicated unconditionally on April 6, 1814.

His conquerors agreed to let him rule the island of Elba off the coast of Tuscany, a mountainous and poor place only eighteen miles long and twelve wide, with some twelve thousand inhabitants. He attacked its problems with characteristic gusto: he arranged for farmers to grow new crops, built new roads and ships, developed iron mines, collected trash rotting in the streets, issued new laws, and revamped the educational system. But after ten months, Napoleon easily escaped with some seven hundred men. He landed in the south of France and swept north as regiments deserted the king and flocked to the emperor's banner. On March 20, 1815, Napoleon arrived in Paris. King Louis XVIII had fled, Napoleon noticed in disgust.

After ruling again for three months, on June 18, 1815, Napoleon's luck ran out once and for all at the Battle of Waterloo in Belgium. After suffering heavy losses, he was completely routed. In Paris, he found that the French people had turned against him. Fearing Louis XVIII would shoot him, Napoleon surrendered to the British, hoping, somewhat naively, that they would give him a farm in England and let him live as a private gentleman.

The British weren't sure what to do with him, though giving him a farm in Wiltshire certainly wasn't on the menu. Finally, they decided to exile Napoleon to the tiny island of St. Helena—ten miles long and five wide—so far away from anything that it would be virtually impossible for him to escape. He was permitted to choose three officers and a dozen servants to accompany him. None of his relatives, whom he had enriched and made monarchs, volunteered to join him.

When, after a sea voyage lasting seventy-one days, his ship dropped anchor in the little port of Jamestown, one of the women on board was heard to say "The devil must have shit this island as he flew from one world to the other." Army surgeon Walter Henry said St. Helena was "the ugliest and most dismal rock conceivable of rugged and splintered surface, rising like an enormous black wart from the face of the deep." The island was a port of call for ships traveling to India or South Africa to take on freshwater and supplies. In 1815, it had a population of four thousand, including a garrison of one thousand men. Napoleon's flotilla brought an additional two thousand soldiers to guard him. His new home, Longwood House, was a sprawling, one-story building of pale yellow stucco and twenty-three rooms. About fifty people lived there, including Napoleon's servants and British guards.

Now his biggest enemy wasn't the Duke of Wellington or the czar of Russia; it was the stultifying boredom. Though he had brought one thousand five hundred books with him, he remarked that he needed sixty thousand to keep him occupied. Up to six hours a day, he dictated his memoirs to a secretary. Every evening at eight, a servant in an embroidered green coat and black silk knee breeches announced, "His Majesty's dinner is served." Napoleon, his aides, and their wives sat down to a formal dinner on silver platters and Sèvres china. Periodically, a giant rat skittered across the room as the diners politely ignored it. After dinner, everyone played cards. Then they listened as Napoleon relived his greatest battles or read out loud. If he managed to stay up until eleven, he would say, "Another victory over time."

Throughout his life, Napoleon had enjoyed excellent health. He exercised regularly, drank alcohol in moderation, and scrubbed himself in a hot bath every morning. Perhaps his wisest step in staying healthy, however, was keeping far away from doctors. Whenever he met a physician, his first question was invariably, "Monsieur, how many patients have you killed in your practice?" He rarely, if ever, took medication or submitted to bleeding, purging, and puking.

His first year on St. Helena, Napoleon was allowed to ride around the island and walk into the port of Jamestown, conversing freely with those he met. But in October 1816, the British governor, Sir Hudson Lowe, heard that American Bonapartists—Napoleon's brother, Joseph, was living in Bordentown, New Jersey—were launching an expedition to rescue him. Fearful and suspicious, Lowe fretted day and night about the dishonor he would suffer if the most important prisoner in the history of the world escaped on his watch. He placed more and more insulting restrictions on his prisoner.

Napoleon soon grew to despise his captor and, for his personal amusement, decided to wage another war, this time on Governor Lowe. When Lowe ordered his men to do a visual check on Napoleon twice a day, the emperor refused to leave his rooms. He drew the blinds whenever he saw a red uniform in the garden. When working in his garden, Napoleon instructed his servants to wear clothing identical to his own, including a huge floppy hat so Lowe's soldiers had no idea which one, if any, was the prisoner. He had his priest, a man of Napoleon's physique, wear his coat and hat and sit with his back to the window, then turn around grinning to show the officer creeping through the garden that he wasn't Napoleon.

Governor Lowe insisted on calling his prisoner General Bonaparte. Napoleon refused to respond to anything spoken or written that did not address him as emperor, sending back the governor's letters unopened. When Lowe sent a case of wine to Longwood House, Napoleon returned it, indicating he suspected the good governor had poisoned it. This new war, with its daily skirmishes and small victories, amused Napoleon. In the interminable tedium, he now had something to live for—torturing Hudson Lowe.

St. Helena was, British pretensions to the contrary, an unhealthful place. The climate was damp and clammy, and the wallpaper of Longwood was often coated with greenish mold. Even worse, Lowe restricted Napoleon's movements, insisting that British officers accompany him riding or walking outside Longwood. Refusing to be guarded by babysitters in red coats, Napoleon stopped riding and walking. With the sudden cessation of exercise, he rapidly gained weight and began to suffer swollen feet, headaches, bleeding gums, and a cough.

On September 20, 1817, for the first time he complained of a dull pain in the area of the torso roughly parallel to his right elbow. From that day forward, other than a period of remission from October 1819 to June 1820, he was never completely free from the symptoms, which included nausea, vomiting, sleeplessness, constipation, and depression. In July 1820, he grew fatigued from the slightest exertion. His pulse was irregular, his hands and feet freezing cold. By the spring of 1821, he could no longer walk without assistance and could barely eat, merely sucking the juice out of meat. The pain in his right side had spread over his entire abdomen.

Though Napoleon had arrived on the island rather fit and gained weight when he stopped exercising, he had lost at least twenty pounds in a few months. When his Italian doctor, François Carlo Antommarchi, urged him to take medications, Napoleon snorted, "Keep your medicines, I don't want to have two diseases, the one I have already and the one you'll give me."

On April 2, he told his English physician, Archibald Arnott, "I have here a sharp pain that, when I feel it, is like being cut with a razor; do you think the pylorus [the bottom of the stomach connected to the duodenum] is affected? My father died of that. Is it not hereditary?" In 1785, the physician who performed Carlo Buonaparte's autopsy had found in the stomach a "tumor of semi-cartilaginous consistency, which was of the shape and size of a large potato or a large elongated pear." But Dr. Arnott reassured him that it was merely gas, and if he took his medication it would go away. The emperor refused.

When Napoleon wrote in his will on April 15 that he was being assassinated by a hired killer of the English oligarchy, it is likely that he knew very well he was dying of stomach cancer but wanted to cause massive difficulties for that archvillain, Governor Lowe. Indeed, Napoleon kept his sense of humor until the end. "I'm not afraid of dying," he said. "The only thing I am afraid of is that the English will keep my body and put it in Westminster Abbey."

By the end of April, he was delirious and vomiting material that looked like coffee grounds, a sign of what we now know to be gastrointestinal bleeding. Periodically, he fell into a coma. On April 26, he saw his beloved Josephine, who had died of pneumonia seven years earlier. "She told me that we were about to see each other again," he said, "never more to part; she assured me that—did you see her?"

On the night of May 4, he mumbled about France, the army, and Josephine. The following day, he fell into a coma and died at the age of fifty-one.

CONTEMPORARY POSTMORTEM

Louis Marchand, the emperor's faithful valet who had been by his side every day on St. Helena, washed the body with eau de cologne and, with two assistant valets, laid it out on a trestle table in the billiard room where the emperor had studied maps. This was, perhaps, the most important autopsy ever performed. At three in the afternoon, Dr. Antommarchi, in the presence of seven other surgeons, all British, and ten French followers of Napoleon, sliced open the body.

The postmortem report stated, "An ulcer which penetrated the coats of the stomach was discovered one inch from the pylorus sufficient to allow the passage of the little finger. The internal surface of the stomach to nearly its whole extent was a mass of cancerous disease, or scirrhous [hard tumorous] portions advancing to cancer, this was particularly noticed near the pylorus . . . The stomach was found nearly filled with a large quantity of fluid, resembling coffee grounds."

Months earlier, Napoleon's stomach ulcer had burst open, causing a hole through which a man could fit his finger. But his liver had glued itself to his stomach, acting as a kind of cork and preventing the stomach acids and food from flooding his body and killing him within hours, as it had Henrietta, duchesse d'Orléans, a century and a half earlier. Though his rupture had sealed, the ulcer developed into cancer. Modern research has shown that untreated gastric ulcers become malignant in about 6 to 9 percent of cases.

Napoleon was buried in his favorite spot on St. Helena, a tranquil grove, but in 1840, he was exhumed in preparation for his return to France. Oddly, though his uniform had decayed, the emperor's body was perfectly preserved, and he looked as if he were sleeping, which many believed was a sign of arsenic poisoning.

MODERN DIAGNOSIS

In the 1960s, a Swedish dentist and Napoleon buff, Dr. Sten Forshufvud, studied Napoleon's illness and recognized twenty-two out of thirty symptoms of arsenic poisoning. Though the French were reluctant to lift the thirty-five tons of highly polished porphyry covering their emperor in Les Invalides in Paris and submit the body to testing, Dr. Forshufvud found numerous locks of Napoleon's hair from his time on St. Helena. Over the years, Napoleon's staff, residents, and visitors had begged for them. When he died, his valet, Marchand, had shaved his head and made many more gifts of Napoleon's hair.

Dr. Forshufvud obtained strands of hair from a variety of sources and submitted them for testing, which revealed arsenic content up to one hundred times the normal amount—proof of poisoning, he believed. But since Dr. Forshufvud's research, Napoleon's hair from his pre–St. Helena days has been tested by research institutes around the world, going back to his earliest years in Corsica. Always, he had arsenic levels about one hundred times normal. So did his first wife, Josephine, and his son, Napoleon II.

While his wife and son may have consumed medications with arsenic and, in the case of Josephine, used arsenic-based cosmetics, Napoleon kept well clear of physicians. A stickler for hygiene, it is possible that since childhood he used an arsenic-based hair tonic to prevent lice infestations. Curiously, his levels did not rise on St. Helena, even though his moldy green wallpaper contained arsenic, and every breeze sent bits of arsenic dust into the air.

In his last, painful months, Napoleon often wondered out loud whether Europe would sink back into the crushing injustices of its past without him, or if the progress and freedom he had brought would, in some form, remain. Would the people, accustomed now to liberty and equality as basic human rights, give them up so easily to returning monarchs? The answer was no, as the revolutions in the decades after his death would prove. Most of all, his legacy lives on in the Napoleonic Code, one of the few documents that has influenced the entire world.

PART III

Poison
IN THE
Modern Era

23

SCIENTIFIC ADVANCES in the VICTORIAN AGE

After the death of Napoleon in 1821, suspicions of royal poison-ing dwindled to almost nothing. One reason was that there was a corresponding dwindling of royal power and less reason to kill a king. In England starting in 1689, and in other European nations after the Napoleonic Wars, the king could no longer snap his fingers and command that a head be separated from its body. Nor could he raise taxes, spend them, and wage war on a whim. Kings no longer ruled. Constitutional monarchs reigned, while parliaments held the true power.

Moreover, advances in medical equipment helped determine what illness a patient had or, in an autopsy, what he had died of. The most basic tools used in doctors' offices today are rather recent inventions. The first stethoscope was invented in 1816 by Paris physician René Theophile Hyacinthe Laënnec, not in the interests of science but of decorum. He had been using his hands to determine the heartbeat and the working of the lungs but was suddenly confronted with a patient in the form of a pretty teenage girl with large breasts. Given the unseem-liness of the situation, he rolled up a piece of paper to listen through and was shocked at how much better he could hear what was going on in her chest. He then created a long wooden tube that he placed against one ear. In 1851, an Irish physician named Arthur Leared invented a stethoscope for both ears.

While court physicians understood that measuring fever was important in understanding the course of a disease, they had no means of doing so. In 1612, a Venetian physician who reveled in the name of Santorio Santorio invented a thermometer that was placed in a patient's mouth. But it was huge, highly unreliable, and took forever to get a reading. It wasn't until 1867 that an English physician, Sir Thomas Allbutt, invented a reliable and accurate thermometer to measure a patient's temperature. It was six inches long and took only five minutes to get an accurate reading.

Until English physician William Harvey's 1628 book *On the Motion of the Heart and Blood,* blood circulation was not understood. Ironically, Harvey's earth-shattering discovery—that the heart pumped blood to the brain and throughout the body—almost ruined his career. People laughed at him in the street, and many stopped coming to his London practice. Though Harvey's theories on blood circulation gradually came to be accepted, a means of measuring blood pressure wasn't available until Austrian physician Samuel Siegfried Karl von Basch invented the sphygmomanometer—the blood pressure cuff—in 1867.

Additionally, chemistry—which for centuries had been hocus-pocus alchemistry—came fully into its own as a modern branch of science. Starting in the mid-eighteenth century, tests were developed to determine the presence of arsenic, though they were often unreliable, depending on what other chemicals were in the mix. Then, in 1833, a British chemist named James Marsh analyzed human organs and leftover coffee in the trial of John Bodle, who was charged with poisoning his nasty, miserly grandfather so he could inherit. A pharmacist testified that he had sold Bodle white arsenic. Marsh performed the usual test in which he mashed up the dead man's organs and the unused coffee and passed bubbling hydrogen sulfide gas through them. The result was the yellow precipitate of arsenic sulfide—proof of poisoning. But by the time Marsh showed his findings at the trial, the precipitate had deteriorated and could no longer be used as evidence. Bodle got off on reasonable doubt.

Marsh, however, knew he was guilty—and, indeed, twenty years later, Bodle admitted he had poisoned the old man. Frustration fueled Marsh's determination to develop a new arsenic test that would hold up in court. By 1836, he perfected what has come to be known as the Marsh test. He added either sulfuric acid or hydrochloric acid to the test sample and then zinc. The mixture of acid and zinc generated hydrogen, and any arsenic in the sample bonded with the hydrogen to form arsine gas, which bubbled out of the solution. The gas passed out of a glass tube, igniting as it escaped through the nozzle and leaving a black precipitate on a sheet of glass next to the flame. The test could detect the slightest trace of arsenic—two parts per million. With a few modifications over the years, the Marsh test was used until the 1970s. In the years after its introduction, scientists developed effective tests for all manner of poison, including alkaloid poisoning, from plants, in 1851. With these scientific advances, dead men told plenty of tales.

In the Victorian era, the microscope propelled medicine forward by leaps and bounds, though it had had a long and unusual history by that time. In 1609, the astronomer Galileo Galilei invented the microscope with far greater magnification than the amplifying lenses that had been around for centuries. Ironically, the individual who truly enhanced the microscope wasn't a scientist, but a cloth merchant. The Dutch draper Anthony van Leeuwenhoek wanted to see the quality of thread better than he could with the magnifying lenses then available. He developed his own lenses but didn't limit himself to studying cloth for his shop. When his curiosity propelled him to examine pond water under a microscope, the draper was shocked to see tiny "animalcules," as he called them, merrily swimming around. His letter to the Royal Society of London is the first record of anyone having seen bacteria.

The Royal Society, alas, didn't take him seriously. On October 20, 1676, Henry Oldenburg, the society secretary, replied, "Your letter of October 10th has been received here with amusement. Your account of myriad 'little animals' seen swimming in rainwater, with the aid of your so-called 'microscope,' caused the members of the society considerable merriment when read at our most recent meeting. Your novel descriptions of the sundry anatomies and occupations of these invisible creatures led one member to imagine that your 'rainwater' might have contained an ample portion of distilled spirits—imbibed by the investigator." Oldenburg continued, "For myself, I withhold judgment as to the sobriety of your observations and the veracity of your instrument. However, a vote having been taken among the members (accompanied, I regret to inform you, by considerable giggling) it has been decided not to publish your communication in the Proceedings of this esteemed society. However, all here wish your 'little animals' health, prodigality and good husbandry by their ingenious 'discoverer.' "

A year later, however, the society arranged for several men to visit Leeuwenhoek. They, too, saw the little swimming animalcules, vindicating him.

After studying pond water, Leeuwenhoek became fascinated with his own saliva and scrapings of plaque between his teeth. On September 17, 1683, he wrote the Royal Society, "I then most always saw, with great wonder, that in the said matter there were many very little living animalcules, very prettily a-moving." In the mouth of an old man who had never cleaned his teeth in his life, Leeuwenhoek found "an unbelievably great company of living animalcules . . . Moreover, the other animalcules were in such enormous numbers, that all the water . . . seemed to be alive." Unfortunately, it took another two hundred years for anyone to question whether such tiny amusing creatures could actually be killers.

By the 1830s, the murderous remedies of bleeding, purging, and puking had fallen out of favor, but it wasn't until the 1870s that the nonsense theories of the four humors and excremental miasmas were tossed into the medical waste bin of history. This progress was mostly due to the work of a German pathologist, Rudolph Virchow, an avid user of the microscope. He replaced humoral theory with cellular doctrine—that disease is caused by changes in the body's cells.

Researchers suddenly made huge strides. In 1876, German physician Robert Koch discovered the first epidemic-causing bacterium: anthrax. A French physician, André Yersin, discovered the bubonic plague bacillus, named *Yersinia pestis* after him, in 1894. In 1880, a French physician named Charles Louis Alphonse Laveran identified the malaria parasite, but it wasn't until 1898 that British surgeon Sir Ronald Ross proved that mosquitoes transmitted the parasite.

New procedures resulted in clear, accurate diagnoses of most illnesses and causes of death. The ignorance-fueled fear that spread rumors of poison was quieted by science.

24

The DEMOCRATIZATION of POISON

Ironically, as nineteenth-century advances in medicine and science reduced the fear of poisoning in royal circles, poisons became much more prevalent in society as a whole. For one thing, they were far more affordable. A murderer no longer had to be rich as a Medici with his own poison factory to do in his enemy. Arsenic rat poison—an unlabeled white powder that looked much like flour or confectioner's sugar—was available for pennies. No laws required the seller to record who bought it. Even children could do so.

The arsenic-based medications that drove King George III mad—James's Powder and Fowler's Solution—were used as home remedies until the 1950s. Arsenic was still used in salves and enemas and inhaled as vapor. Treatments for syphilis switched from mercury to arsenic in 1908 with a new medication called Salvarsan, which was used until penicillin became available to the general public in 1945.

Because of industrialization, poisonous cosmetics, which had previously been the luxuries of the rich and noble, became affordable to the working class. Cosmetics containing large dollops of mercury, arsenic, lead, and other harmful substances were no longer just for queens and countesses; even commoners could buy them. In the 1860s, a skin whitening lotion called Laird's Bloom of Youth, which had been advertised as a "delightful and harmless toilet preparation," was found to cause paralysis, weight loss, nausea, headaches, and palsy due to its high levels of lead acetate. Many other skin care products contained mercury, lead, carbolic acid, and other poisonous ingredients. Berry's Freckle Ointment contained mercuric chloride. Dr. MacKenzie's Improved Harmless Arsenic Wafer speaks for itself.

Poison invaded the sphere of middle-class home décor and clothing. In 1775, German chemist Karl Scheele made a brilliant green pigment from copper arsenite—Scheele green—that became immediately popular for wallpaper, including that used in Napoleon's residence on St. Helena. In 1814, chemists in the German city of Schweinfurt developed Schweinfurt green, which was produced in a variety of hues and made from copper acetate and copper arsenite. Green, all of it arsenic-based, became the most fashionable color of the nineteenth century, wildly popular for clothing, furniture, paints, soap, food coloring, upholstery, drapes, and children's toys, resulting in countless deaths.

In 1864, a scientist found that the arsenic in the wallpaper of an average-sized living room was enough to kill a hundred people. Children, in particular, sickened and sometimes died in rooms with green wallpaper. In 1858, arsenic wallpaper covered more than a million square miles of walls in British homes. By the 1880s, when people realized the dangers and had the stuff removed, the wallpaper removers often fainted from the arsenic fumes. Homeowners had to open the windows and resuscitate the men with brandy. But just removing the wallpaper wasn't enough. The homeowner would also have to replace the green Venetian blinds that threw off arsenic dust each time they were opened or closed. And reupholster all the furniture. And get new carpets. And lampshades.

And clothing. A London physician analyzed cloth for a ball gown made of Scheele's green and found more than sixty grains of arsenic per yard of fabric, loosely adhered. Considering that a gown over a hoop skirt required more than twenty yards of fabric, the dress contained some one thousand grains of arsenic, enough to poison more than two hundred people. While the belle of the ball was swirling and dipping, she was spraying the air with arsenic dust. She was, quite literally, drop-dead gorgeous.

In one London ballet, the dancers were poisoned by their green water-nymph costumes. We can envision them halting mid-pirouette to rush offstage to vomit. Seamstresses and others who worked with poisonous material frequently became ill. In 1861, nineteen-year-old Matilda Sheurer, who dusted artificial flowers for gowns and headdresses with arsenic powder, died after months of alarming symptoms. Her eyeballs and fingernails turned green, and she vomited, convulsed, and foamed at the mouth. Her autopsy found arsenic in her stomach, liver, and lungs.

Even today, museum curators working with green nineteenth-century clothing wear masks and gloves to avoid inhaling the arsenic dust that floats off them when they are moved.

Arsenic was mixed with wax to give candles a smooth surface and sheen. When the candle burned, arsenic was released into the air. In the era before pesticides, the ever-present problem of flies was solved by using arsenic-saturated flypaper. The poisoned flies kamikazed their way into people's beer, and even if they were immediately fished out, the beer made people throw up. Farmers soaked their wheat seed in an arsenic solution to protect against parasitic infestations. Grocers shined fruit with it. Brewers used arsenic glucose in their beer.

Thus the Marsh test was no longer as useful as James Marsh had hoped it would be in convicting a murderer. Not only could the poison have been mistaken for sugar and put in the victim's tea, but with arsenic ever-present in Victorian society, the victim could have absorbed, inhaled, or ingested it quite innocently.

While royals, too, suffered along with the common man from poisonous cosmetics, medications, and ornaments, their hygiene, at least, improved greatly in the Victorian era. Regular bathing became increasingly popular as the nineteenth century progressed, and most palaces and stately homes had running water and flush toilets by the 1880s. Gone were the overflowing chamber pots and the germs that came with them.

And, if doctors couldn't heal many illnesses, at least they had stopped actively killing their patients. Mortality was reduced and diagnosis improved. Members of royal courts, who in past centuries had seen poison lurking behind every illness, could finally relax.

25

MODERN MEDICIS

The REBIRTH *of* POLITICAL POISON

These days, those who publicly oppose Russia's president Vladimir Putin must eye their food and drink with as much concern as any Renaissance king. But instead of waving a unicorn horn over their dining table to detect poison, Russian dissidents would be well advised to use a Geiger counter. Knowing that karma is a bitch, Putin is the only world leader known to employ a personal food tester as the kings of old did. Rather than relying on his security team to ensure his food is free of poison, as other leaders do, he has a physician on his staff who works closely with his personal chef. Both ingest a bit of everything well before it is served to him. We can picture them crossing their fingers that they won't vomit, pass out, and glow an eerie green in the dark.

Russian assassins have developed toxic materials truly worthy of a nuclear superpower, cooking up new radioactive poisons that cause massive organ failure. Some of these poisons elude even the most advanced tests to identify them, bringing us full circle with the Renaissance, when physicians had no way of determining what kind of poison had been used to kill the patient, if any.

Throughout its tumultuous history, Russia has seen its fair share of political assassinations. One infamous murder at the tail end of the imperial period—when poison had become the stuff of dusty history

243

tomes at other European courts—was that of the mad monk Gregory Rasputin. In 1916, palace conspirators—jealous of Rasputin's influence over Emperor Nicholas II and Empress Alexandra—reportedly gave him enough cyanide-laced wine and cakes to kill an elephant. Rasputin only complained of a tickling in his throat, probably because he had been taking a theriac to build up his resistance to poisons, so they had to shoot him.

In 1921, the Soviets established their first laboratory—the *Kamera*—for the manufacture of poisons. Their goal was to develop odorless, tasteless, and colorless poisons that victims could not detect when ingesting and would leave no trace. Whenever a poison was detected in the corpse of a political activist, it would not be used again. For this reason, the *Kamera* constantly developed new poisons. The Soviets tested them on condemned prisoners, just as the sixteenth-century Medicis did in their *fonderie* in the Palazzo Vecchio, but the Soviet victims were mostly political enemies. Recent events have shown that this laboratory did not disappear with communism in 1991 but still exists. According to Boris Volodarsky, a former Russian military-intelligence agent and author of the 2009 book *Inside the KGB's Poison Factory*, doctors at the *Kamera* calculate a victim's height, weight, eating habits, and other information in order to select a poison. The optimal dose is one that will kill the target but leave no trace, resulting in a coroner's verdict of death by natural or undetermined causes.

The Russians have put the knowledge gained from their poison lab to good use over the nearly one hundred years since its inception. In 1936, the Communist leader of Russia's Abkhaz region, forty-three-year-old Nestor Lakoba, was poisoned over dinner by his political rival Lavrentiy Beria. The official cause of death? Heart attack. After a solemn state funeral, Beria reportedly had Lakoba's body dug up and burned so no one could ever discover the true cause of death. In 1938, Abram Aronovich Slutsky, head of the Soviet foreign intelligence service, was allegedly killed by a political enemy with hydrocyanic acid–laced tea and cakes. Official cause of death? Heart attack.

The brilliant Nikolai Konstantinovich Koltsov, an early innovator in the field of genetics, proposed in 1927 that traits were passed from one generation to the next by means of a "giant hereditary molecule" consisting of "two mirror strands that would replicate in a semi-conservative fashion using each strand as a template"—in other words, DNA, which was confirmed in 1953. When the strongly independent scientist refused to change his findings to fit the party line, his enemies accused him of promoting Hitlerian racist propaganda. Koltsov was poisoned in 1940, though doctors called it a stroke. His wife committed suicide the same day.

Two Ukrainian political activities—Lev Rebet in 1957 and Stepan Andriyovych Bandera in 1959—were shot in the face with a jet of cyanide gas from a crushed capsule. The poison made the deaths look like heart attacks. But the assassin, Bohdan Stashynsky, defected to the West two years later and confessed to both murders.

POISON AT THE PINNACLE

Even the Kremlin's top leaders may have been poisoned. In 2012, doctors at the University of Maryland's annual clinico-pathological conference concluded that the founder of Russian communism, Vladimir Lenin, died in 1924 after being poisoned by his political successor, Joseph Stalin. Lenin had already had several strokes, but he was recovering nicely. Within a couple of hours after a friend of Stalin's visited Lenin, he suffered violent convulsions—a symptom more in line with poisoning than stroke—and died. The autopsy physician found that Lenin's cerebral arteries were so calcified that when he tapped them with tweezers they sounded like stone, which would have indicated he had been ripe for a stroke. Yet the Soviet government ordered that no toxicology tests be performed on Lenin, though they were routinely carried out on other deceased leaders.

What goes around comes around. A recent investigation indicates that Joseph Stalin, the brutal leader of the Soviet Union, may have died from poison instead of his reported stroke in 1953. Early accounts of his autopsy revealed that he had suffered extensive stomach bleeding, a symptom of warfarin, a tasteless and colorless medication that is poisonous in high doses. Any mention of stomach bleeding was removed from his official medical report. The guests at Stalin's last dinner included Georgy Malenkov, who briefly succeeded Stalin, and Nikita Khrushchev, who succeeded Malenkov. Another diner was Lavrentiy

Beria, chief of the secret police, who had poisoned Nestor Lakoba back in 1936. In his memoirs, Khrushchev wrote that Beria boasted of killing Stalin.

One of the most notorious Russian poison assassinations was that of Georgi Markov, an anti-communist Bulgarian writer. On the morning of September 7, 1978, the forty-nine-year-old was waiting for a bus on London's Waterloo Bridge when someone poked him in the back of his right thigh with an umbrella. The heavily built man mumbled an apology and stepped into a cab. Markov soon developed a fever and checked himself into the hospital that evening. He died four days later. Forensic pathologists found in his thigh a pellet the size of a pinhead with traces of ricin. The pellet had been coated in wax, which was designed to melt at the temperature of a human body, slowly releasing the poison into the bloodstream. British investigations revealed that the Bulgarian secret police had worked with the Soviet KGB to plan and execute the hit.

One of the most creative Russian political poisonings involved a lethal lamp. Anatoly Sobchak was a politician best known for his tenure as the flamboyant mayor of St. Petersburg from 1991 to 1996. His trusted deputy and mentee was Vladimir Putin. In 1999, Sobchak strongly supported Putin's run for president, but his support wasn't necessarily a good thing. He called Putin "the new Stalin," and though he meant it as a compliment, Putin wasn't thrilled. Sobchak also reminisced fondly to journalists about a young Vladimir, relating events that Putin had edited out of his official life story.

On February 17, 2000, Putin met with Sobchak and asked him to leave immediately for the city of Kaliningrad to campaign for him. Sobchak, accompanied by two bodyguards, obediently did so. On February 20, he apparently died of a heart attack. In a striking coincidence, his young, physically fit bodyguards also had heart attacks at the same time. They survived, however, and were treated for symptoms of poisoning. A Russian forensics expert believed that someone had sprayed poison onto the reading lamp next to Sobchak's bed. The heat from the lamp would have vaporized the poison throughout the room, killing its intended victim, who was sitting right next to it, and only sickening the guards who may have stuck their heads in to say goodnight. The vapor would have completely dissipated over time, leaving no trace.

The case of Emir Khattab gives new meaning to the term "poison pen letter." Khattab, born in Saudi Arabia in 1967 as Thamir Saleh Abdullah, left home at eighteen to fight against the Soviet invasion of Afghanistan, where he lost the fingers of his right hand while making a bomb. He fought with Islamic insurgents in Azerbaijan, Tajikistan, Bosnia, Dagestan, and Chechnya, becoming a rich warlord.

In 1999, a series of Russian apartment building bombings killed 293 and injured more than 1,000. The FSB—the renamed and only slightly remodeled version of the Soviet KGB—blamed the bombings on Khattab, and the groundswell of patriotic outrage not only propelled Putin to power but gave him an excuse to invade Chechnya again, beginning the Second Chechen War. Khattab denied any role in the bombings but boasted of inflicting devastating losses on Russian forces in Chechnya. His meticulously planned ambushes in narrow gorges killed dozens of Russian soldiers, and his frontal attacks and homemade antipersonnel mines may have killed hundreds more.

The FSB, aware of Khattab's thorough measures to prevent assassination, came up with a clever means of killing him. They placed two men in Khattab's group who proved useful in transferring money, buying weapons, and delivering mail. Though wary at first, over time Khattab came to trust them. The double agents picked up his mail from a post office box in Azerbaijan; he looked forward to a monthly missive from his mother in Saudi Arabia. After working for Khattab for a year, the men intercepted a letter from an Islamic fighter from a nearby country, doused it with poison—probably sarin—sealed it back up again, and delivered it to Khattab on March 20, 2002.

The warlord took the envelope into his tent and opened it. According to sources in the Russian special services, "He came out a half hour later with his face pale, rubbing his face with the stump of his arm, and then he fell into the arms of his bodyguards." Then, feeling better, he instructed his men to release the couriers, whom they had been holding. But after their departure, Khattab "fell into some bushes, and a moment later he was dead." Two months later, one of the couriers, a man named Ibragim, was found dead with five bullets in the head.

Sarin attacks the central nervous system, shutting down the lungs. Khattab would have died as a result of asphyxia. Those earlier would-be assassins who hoped to kill Pope Alexander VI in 1499 and King

Louis XIV in 1679 with poison-drenched letters would have been quite impressed.

Fifty-three-year-old Yuri Petrovich Shchekochikhin, a Russian member of parliament and an investigative journalist, believed it was not Emir Khattab, the terrorist, who had orchestrated the devastating apartment building bombings that killed 293 Russians in 1999. Shchekochikhin believed the mastermind was none other than Vladimir Putin, who used the bombings to manipulate the Russian people into supporting his invasion of Chechnya. Shchekochikhin was a member of the independent commission formed to investigate the bombings, which closed down when the government refused to respond to requests for information.

While investigating money-laundering activities of FSB officers through the Bank of New York, Shchekochikhin learned that the FBI was conducting a similar investigation and set up a meeting with them to share information. But just before he left for the United States, he ate something that disagreed with him and died. His medical documents have been "classified" by the Russian authorities. His relatives were denied an official medical report about the cause of his illness and were forbidden to take specimens of his tissues for an independent medical investigation. Some of his journalist friends managed to smuggle out tissue samples during his sixteen-day illness and sent them to foreign specialists, who were unable to conclude what killed him. However, the symptoms of his illness fit a pattern of poisoning by radioactive materials.

POISONOUS POLITICAL CUISINE

Fifty-year-old Viktor Yushchenko, a 2004 Ukrainian presidential candidate, was heavily pro-West, leaning away from Russia and toward NATO, political freedom, and fighting corruption. His opponent in the race, Viktor Yanukovych, was closely allied with Russia. On September 5, in the final weeks of a bitter and sometimes violent campaign, Yushchenko ate soup with a group of senior Ukrainian officials and almost immediately became deathly ill.

He was flown to a Viennese hospital where doctors found he had acute pancreatitis, chloracne in his face, which became swollen and pockmarked, and a serious viral infection. They also discovered in

Yushchenko's blood levels of TCCD, a chemical compound also known as dioxin, 6,000 times above normal, though they estimated he had had 50,000 times the normal amount soon after consuming the poison. First created in the late nineteenth century as a by-product of the burning of organic materials, TCCD is odorless and tasteless. An ingredient in Agent Orange, it is 170,000 times more poisonous than cyanide.

Doctors agree that Yushchenko rid himself immediately of much of the poison by vomiting and diarrhea. Ironically, the disfiguring lumps on his face may have also helped save his life. Some of the dioxin was isolated in the tumors, far away from the liver and other vital organs.

In August 2009, the respected British medical journal *The Lancet* published a paper by Swiss and Ukrainian researchers on Yushchenko's case, concluding that the poison "was so pure that it was definitely made in a laboratory."

When the victim pointed the finger at Russia for poisoning him, the Russians accused him of either working with doctors to falsify his records or poisoning himself in an effort to win sympathy and votes. When one of his dinner companions, the former deputy chief of Ukraine's security service, Volodymyr Satsyuk, fled to Russia, the Russian government granted him Russian citizenship to protect him from extradition. Yushchenko won the presidential election, though it took years of medical treatment for his face to resume something approaching his former good looks. He said, "I fell foul of Ukraine's political cuisine, which it seems can kill."

A NICE HOT CUP OF TEA

In September 2004, forty-four-year-old journalist and Putin critic Anna Politkovskaya was hoping to cover breaking news; Islamic terrorists had taken over a school in the city of Beslan, in Russia's autonomous North Caucasus region, and were holding some one thousand people hostage. Waiting in a Moscow airport along with many other journalists hoping to fly to Beslan, Politkovskaya realized that all the flights to Beslan were being canceled.

Then a man claiming to be an airport executive approached her and said he could get her on a flight. When she boarded a minibus to get to the plane, the driver told her the FSB had arranged for her to join the flight. It is surprising she didn't tell the driver to turn around and take her back to the airport. The FSB was no friend of Politkovskaya, an investigative journalist who often uncovered unsavory stories about Russia's leaders. Certainly she shouldn't have consumed anything offered by a flight attendant.

"I ask for a tea . . . ," she wrote in a newspaper article. "At 21:50 I drink it. At 22:00 I realize that I have to call the air stewardess as I am rapidly losing consciousness. My other memories are scrappy: the stewardess weeps and shouts: 'We're landing, hold on!' "

When Politkovskaya woke in a hospital, a nurse bending over her whispered that she had been brought in "almost hopeless." Then the nurse added, "My dear, they tried to poison you." The journalist reported that all the blood and urine samples had been destroyed, as per "orders from on high," according to the doctors. In a 2004 book, *Putin's Russia*, she wrote, "We are hurtling back into a Soviet abyss, into an information vacuum that spells death from our own ignorance. All we have left is the internet, where information is still freely available. For the rest, if you want to go on working as a journalist, it's total servility to Putin. Otherwise, it can be death, the bullet, poison, or trial—whatever our special services, Putin's guard dogs, see fit."

A downside to poison—whether it's arsenic or a more recently developed toxin—is the uncertainty of its efficacy. Much as the Roman emperor Nero, impatient with trying to poison his objectionable mother, finally had her stabbed, the Russians, too, were unwilling to fiddle with another cup of tea for Anna Politkovskaya. Her enemies arranged for her to be shot as she stood holding bags of groceries in the elevator of her Moscow apartment building. Five men have been convicted of carrying out the crime, but no one is saying who ordered it. She was murdered on October 7, 2006, which happens to be Putin's birthday.

THE HOTTEST TEA ON THE PLANET

Alexander Litvinenko was a former Russian intelligence officer who fled to Great Britain, where he wrote articles and books highly critical of Vladimir Putin, accusing him of organizing terrorist attacks on Russian soil—including the 1999 apartment bombings—to blame others, incite fear, and increase his power.

On November 1, 2006—two weeks after he accused Putin of ordering the murder of Anna Politkovskaya—Litvinenko met at a London hotel with two former KGB officers, Andrey Lugovoy and Dmitri Kovtun, and later that day fell ill with vomiting and diarrhea. He told doctors he had been poisoned, though extensive tests found no trace of any unusual substances. His blood and urine samples were sent to the UK's Atomic Weapons Establishment, where specialists conducted tests using gamma spectroscopy to find evidence of radioactive poison. They found no signs of radioactivity other than a mysterious small spike. By chance, a doctor who overhead some colleagues discussing the spike had worked for Britain's early atomic bomb program and realized it could indicate the presence of polonium-210. A million times more poisonous than cyanide, this substance emits radioactive particles that tear cells apart, destroying the immune system and causing catastrophic organ failure. Tests showed a staggering amount of polonium-210 in Litvinenko's samples—two hundred times the amount needed to kill him.

Because there had never been a known case of polonium-210 poisoning, the standard battery of poison tests did not look for it. If the doctor had not overheard the conversation, the poison would probably have gone undetected, as the assassins must have hoped. Polonium-210 can be produced only in state-regulated nuclear reactors, and the dose that poisoned Litvinenko has since been traced back to a Russian nuclear power plant. Investigators collecting evidence at the hotel where Litvinenko met with the men found a teapot with off-the-charts levels of polonium. They analyzed the car that had dropped him off at his home—a friend had given him a ride—and decided the vehicle was so radioactive it had to be destroyed. They tested his house and found such high contamination levels that his family couldn't live there for six months.

When he died on November 23, Litvinenko's body was so radioactive it was left in the hospital bed for two days before being moved to cold storage, and doctors waited a week before performing the autopsy in hazmat suits. But one of the assassins ended up poisoning himself. Andrey Lugovoy, who had returned to Russia two days after the poisoning, received hospital treatment for radiation poisoning.

In May 2007, the British government formally asked Russia to extradite Lugovoy to Britain where he would be charged with murder. Russia refused, arguing that its constitution forbids extraditing Russian citizens. Since 2007, Lugovoy has been a member of the Russian Duma, or parliament, and now enjoys parliamentary immunity from any charges. In January 2016, a thorough UK investigation found that Andrey Lugovoy and Dmitri Kovtun had poisoned Litvinenko and had likely been acting under the instructions of the FSB and Vladimir Putin, a finding Russia vehemently denies.

In a stunning display of bad taste, in 2015 Lugovoy's young model wife opened a chain of tea shops in Moscow, though it's hard to imagine she has any customers.

THE PERILS OF SORREL SOUP

Alexander Perepilichny was a Russian national who had sought refuge in the UK while helping a Swiss investigation into a money-laundering scheme, the theft of $230 million from the Russian treasury. In November 2012, the forty-four-year-old felt unwell after lunch and decided to clear his head with a brisk jog around his exclusive, high-security neighborhood outside London. He was found unconscious a hundred feet from his home. The person who found him called an ambulance, but he died thirty minutes later.

Perepilichny had recently had a thorough physical examination in order to take out a multimillion-dollar life insurance policy and was found to be in very good health. Indeed, it was his life insurance company that found evidence of poisoning. The local police had performed routine toxicology tests, all of which had come back negative, and then disposed of the stomach contents. They declared that his death was unsuspicious. But the insurance company, which would not have to pay out if Perepilichny was murdered, hired its own toxicologist, who conducted more extensive tests on minuscule amounts of food still left in the stomach. She found traces of a rare and deadly poison from the gelsemium plant, found only in remote parts of China and loaded with toxins related to strychnine. According to hearsay evidence, Perepilichny had eaten a large bowl of Russian sorrel soup for lunch, and the poisonous plant could easily have been swapped for the sorrel.

At the inquest, the senior coroner requested that the British government turn over information regarding threats on Perepilichny's life and his contacts with certain suspects. The government announced it would not release the information for reasons of national security.

THE DOUBLE WHAMMY

Only one person in the world is known to have survived Kremlin poison twice. The anti-Putin activist Vladimir Kara-Murza lobbied vigorously in Washington for the Magnitsky Act, a US law imposing sanctions on Russians involved in human rights abuses. The law was named after Russian lawyer and accountant Sergei Magnitsky, who had been investigating fraud involving Russian tax officials, was jailed on fake charges, and died in prison from brutal beatings and inadequate medical care in 2009.

President Barack Obama signed the law in December 2012, enraging the Russian government. Kara-Murza's partner in pushing the legislation, Boris Nemtsov, also an outspoken critic of Putin, was shot and killed on February 27, 2015, on a bridge near the Kremlin.

On May 26, 2015, thirty-three-year-old Kara-Murza suddenly became violently ill in Moscow during a meeting, about two hours after eating lunch in a restaurant. He vomited, lost consciousness, and was taken to the hospital. Over the next seventy-two hours, his brain swelled and his lungs, heart, kidneys, liver, and intestines started to shut down. In a coma for a week, he was given a 5 percent chance of survival. Russian doctors cleaned unidentified toxins from his blood with hemodialysis. Against all odds, he survived, though he suffered nerve damage for a year. His wife sent some samples of his blood, hair, and fingernails to a toxicology lab in France, which found traces of heavy metals, dozens of times over the normal amount, but was unable to pinpoint the poison.

Undeterred by the attempt on his life, Kara-Murza continued to live in Moscow and pursue his activism against Kremlin corruption, frequently traveling abroad to speak on the subject. On January 9, 2017, he was delighted when the outgoing Obama administration placed sanctions on General Alexander Bastrykin, a close Putin ally who headed the Russian Investigative Committee, a government agency that has brought trumped-up criminal charges against anti-Putin activists.

Then, on February 2, 2017, Kara-Murza, while staying at his

in-laws' Moscow apartment, suddenly felt the same alarming symptoms—difficulty breathing, a hammering heart, nausea, and vomiting. This time he knew what to do. He went immediately to the same hospital that had successfully treated him the first time, where the same doctor was waiting. He fell into an induced coma as they replaced every drop of blood in his body. This time, the hospital sent samples of Kara-Murza's blood, hair, and fingernails to labs in France and Israel to find the kind of poison used. So far, they have been unable to identify it. His diagnosis is a vague one: acute intoxication by an unidentified substance. It seems to be a new, untraceable poison developed by the *Kamera*.

The activist was released from the hospital February 19, 2017, and traveled to Washington—where his wife and children live—to recuperate. "The doctors say, if there is a third time, that'll be it. I will not survive this again," he said, adding, "I am not brave, just stubborn."

THE STRANGE DEATH OF MR. ARAFAT

Not all recent, mysteriously deceased political figures are Russians. When former Palestinian president Yasser Arafat sat down to his last lunch on October 25, 2004, in his compound in Ramallah, in the West Bank, he was seventy-five and in good health. Outside, Israeli troops continued to enforce a years-long house arrest, claiming Arafat incited violence. Four hours after his meal, Arafat began to suffer vomiting, abdominal pain, and watery diarrhea but no fever—all symptoms of poisoning.

When he died seventeen days later in a Paris hospital of a mysterious infection and possible stroke, rumors abounded of poison. But the hospital destroyed all biological samples it had taken, no autopsy was performed, and the body was not embalmed.

In 2012, the Al Jazeera Media Network conducted a nine-month study of Arafat's death, concluding that none of the medical explanations for rare blood disorders or generalized infections could be correct. The Institute for Radiation Physics at the University of Lausanne in Switzerland found traces of polonium on Arafat's personal belongings kept by his wife, Suha, an indication that he had abnormal levels of polonium in his body at death. Moreover, the institute stated that some 60 to 80 percent of the polonium it found had not come from natural sources. Yet it was not enough evidence to determine a cause of death.

The institute pointed out that Arafat had not lost his hair, as Alexander Litvinenko had when he was poisoned with polonium-210, and some of its findings were not consistent with radiation poisoning. Dr. Ely Karmon, a specialist in chemical, biological, radiological, and nuclear terrorism at Israel's International Institute for Counter-Terrorism, said that given the 138-day half-life of polonium, it would have disintegrated far more over the course of eight years than the studies found. It if had, indeed, originally been so astonishingly high, Arafat's wife should also have been poisoned by staying by his side in the hospital and touching his clothing.

In November 2012, Arafat's body was exhumed and samples given to three different labs. While polonium shows up most clearly in the body's soft tissues, no organs remained, and the labs could only test bones, which would have had a much lower poison content than the spleen, liver, and kidneys. On November 6, 2013, Al Jazeera reported that the Swiss forensic team had found levels of polonium in Arafat's ribs and pelvis eighteen times higher than normal. But Swiss researchers stated that the theory of polonium poisoning was only "moderately supported."

The French lab admitted to finding much higher than normal traces of polonium but decided Arafat had died of natural causes. The Russian lab, too, decreed that there was no evidence of death by polonium poisoning, though the official report showed that of the twenty samples, only those four that were least likely to show polonium exposure were tested.

Into this soup of vagueness, confusion, and backpedaling strode David Barclay, a professor emeritus at Robert Gordon University in Scotland and a veteran forensic investigator specializing in analyzing physical evidence in murder cases. After studying all the reports, he wrote that the average amount of polonium in an individual who has died of natural causes is between 25 and 50 millibecquerels per gram of calcium, a tiny level from the decay of radon naturally occurring in the environment. "Arafat's ribs were around 900 millibecquerels," Barclay pointed out. "That is 18 to 36 times more than the average, even at the time of exhumation. And remember, that took place over eight years later when the polonium-210 had been reduced by twenty-one half-lives. So at the time of his death in 2004, he had over two million times that level circulating in his blood and being deposited in his bones." He added that results showed that the polonium-210 had been manufactured in a nuclear reactor. Clearly, Arafat could not have absorbed it by taking a walk.

Moreover, Barclay stated, the high polonium readings were not the result of postmortem contamination, as they were found in stains from his urine, blood, sweat, and in those bones that have the greatest blood supply. "Toxicologists in general and the Swiss scientists in particular," he wrote, "can never state just from the science that someone definitely has died of, for example, cyanide or strychnine. That is because the person might have then jumped off a bridge, or died under a train, so death due to a poison always depends also on the absence of any other cause being present . . . However, very exhaustive tests were performed by the French Percy Hospital during his final days, without result. Arafat had no other disease, no cancer, and no heart disease."

It is possible that for political reasons the true cause of Yasser Arafat's death will always remain cloaked in mystery.

AN AIRPORT PRANK

It's highly unusual for a political poisoning to occur on security cameras, but that's what happened on February 13, 2017, as Kim Jong-nam, the estranged forty-five-year-old brother of North Korean dictator Kim Jong-un, was walking through the airport in Kuala Lumpur, Malaysia. Suddenly a young woman ran up to him and applied something to his face. Moments later, another one did the same. After they raced off, he began to feel ill and had difficulty breathing. He approached an airline representative and asked her to call an ambulance, but he died about fifteen minutes after the attack en route to the hospital.

After an unseemly tug-of-war over the body—North Korea wanted it handed over immediately, without an autopsy—Malaysian officials who performed the postmortem discovered that Kim had been poisoned by VX, an odorless, tasteless liquid and the most toxic nerve agent ever produced. VX—which stands for "venomous agent X"—is a fast-acting toxin that disrupts the transmission of nerve impulses, leading to respiratory collapse and heart failure. A single drop of the poison is enough to kill an adult, whether it is inhaled or absorbed through the skin.

Experts were astonished that the VX hadn't killed the women who applied it. Then the director of a nonproliferation research program of the Middlebury Institute of International Studies at Monterey suggested that two nonfatal components were mixed together on Kim's face to create VX. Called a binary concoction, it offers safer storage and transportation than the toxin itself. And indeed, according to a police report, one of the women said she was told to spray Kim's face, after which the second woman held a handkerchief over it.

Investigators wanted to discover how VX—a substance banned as a weapon of mass destruction by the 1997 Chemical Weapons Convention—was obtained in Kuala Lumpur. North Korea, however, never signed the treaty and is believed to have VX stockpiled. Malaysian police believe the two separate ingredients were shipped in diplomatic pouches, which are generally not inspected by customs on their entry into a country.

The two women—a twenty-five-year-old Indonesian citizen, Siti Aisyah, and a twenty-eight-year-old Vietnamese citizen, Doan Thi Huong—were charged in the murder. Both reportedly worked in Kuala Lumpur massage parlors. Aisyah claimed to have met a man named James at a popular bar. He presented himself as a producer of a reality TV show, where people are paid to play pranks on unsuspecting individuals in malls, train stations, and hotels. Aisyah reported that she had played several pranks—she said she thought she was spraying baby oil on Kim Jong-nam's face—and James paid her between $100 and $150 each time. James, however, turned out to be a North Korean, thirty-year-old Ri Ji U. The Malaysian police, however, dismissed claims of a prank and believed both women knew they were taking part in an assassination. Four North Koreans that police believe were involved in the attack have returned home.

At first, investigators are uncertain why Kim Jong-un would order a hit on his pudgy, balding brother, who was, after all, a rather pathetic character. Kim Jong-nam, though the oldest son, was never fully accepted by his family. His grandfather, North Korea's founding president, Kim Il-sung, didn't like Kim Jong-nam's mother, an actress, and never approved of her marrying his son and heir, Kim Jong-il. Kim

Jong-nam was shuttled around to relatives in Moscow and a Swiss boarding school, while his father had two more sons with an opera singer. The current ruler, Kim Jong-un, is the younger.

Growing up, it became clear that Kim Jong-nam lacked the killer instinct the next leader required; for instance, he showed an alarming leniency toward defectors. He lost his last chance to become the next dictator in 2001, when he was arrested trying to sneak into Japan on a false passport. During his interrogation, he confessed that he had only wanted to go to Tokyo's Disneyland. As an adult, Kim Jong-nam led a peripatetic life, living recently in Macau under Chinese government protection. He loved to gamble and had, as far as is known, two wives, a mistress, and six children, and traveled aimlessly around visiting them.

Kim Jong-un has ordered the executions of many senior officials, including his uncle, evidently seeing them as threats to his power. But why his older half brother? Why now? And why in full view of security cameras? It turns out that $120,000 in $100 bills was found in Kim Jong-nam's backpack, money which he had apparently recently received during a two-hour meeting with a CIA agent in return for spilling the beans on his tyrant brother. As for the murder of his half brother on video, North Korea's Dear Respected Comrade Leader, as Kim Jong-un is known, clearly wanted the world to see his ruthlessness up close and personal on the evening news. It sent a message far more bone-chilling than the launch of yet another missile whistling over Japan.

Kim Jong-nam had never liked Kim Jong-un. In 2012 he told a journalist that his brother was too young and inexperienced to lead the nation: "Without reforms, North Korea will collapse, and when such changes take place, the regime will collapse."

But it was Kim Jong-nam who collapsed.

The ROYAL ART of LIVING
and DYING

As a historian, I am often asked if I would like to have been a princess, centuries ago. It is a reasonable question as I often decry the mediocrity of modernity. To me, T-shirts, flip-flops, and baseball caps are death by a thousand cuts. I shake my head at the inelegance of strip malls, big-box stores, and traffic jams. On the other hand, I am seduced by beautiful gowns, glittering jewels, and gorgeous palaces. I revel in fantasies of candlelit banquets, river regattas, and royal pageantry.

It should be quite clear, however, that my answer to a theoretical life as a baroque princess is a firm no. At this point, I would be afraid to time travel even for a few hours—attend a Versailles ball, let's say—because I might bring something horrifying back with me. Worms, perhaps. And if I stayed there longer, well, it would be hard to enjoy the splendors of court life if I were in agonizing pain. Or dead.

Nowadays, thanks to advances in medicine, most of us live to grow old—ancient, in fact, by Renaissance standards. Still, we are in no position to be smug. Despite the universal human goal to live a long and healthy life, today our actions and lifestyle curtail our longevity just as those of our ancestors did. Though we might laugh at lead face paint, mercury enemas, and arsenic skin lotions, future generations will certainly laugh at us for poisoning ourselves with chemotherapy and whatever unknown elements in our modern society cause increasingly high rates of cancer, autism, and dementia.

Despite the miracles of modern medicine that extend our lives, at some point our human forms—at once so wondrous and so fragile—will go the way of all flesh. Let us remember the last words of French royal mistress Agnes Sorel, poisoned by mercury in 1450. "It is a little thing," she whispered of her body as her organs shut down, "and soiled, and smelling of our frailty."

But that is never the end of the story. Our art, our music, and our discoveries remain behind, as do the echoes of our beauty, courage, self-sacrifice, and love.

PICK YOUR POISON

Poison, like anything else, has its own fashion cycles. Plant toxins were most popular in the ancient world, whereas modish murderers during the Renaissance and Baroque eras favored heavy metal poisons. Scientific advances in the nineteenth and twentieth centuries have created a new and deadly slate of chemical and radioactive compounds.

HEAVY METAL POISONS

Antimony: a lustrous gray metalloid, found in nature mainly as the sulfide mineral stibnite.

Poisoning symptoms: similar to arsenic poisoning although it is not nearly as deadly. Antimony causes vomiting sooner than arsenic, often before a lethal amount is absorbed into the bloodstream, and for centuries was used as a remedy by physicians hoping to make the patients vomit forth the evil humors causing illness.

Arsenic: a mineral that comes in different colors: gray, black, red—called realgar—and yellow—known as orpiment. Most poisoners used white arsenic, made by heating arsenic ore and crushing it into a white crystalline powder soluble in water and virtually undetectable in food or drink.

Poisoning symptoms: violent vomiting, watery diarrhea, abdominal pain, muscle spasms in the calves, sore mouth and throat, difficulty swallowing, unremitting thirst, weak pulse, cold damp skin, kidney failure, coma, and death.

Lead: a gray metallic ore.

Poisoning symptoms: constipation, weakness, numbness in limbs, water buildup in the brain, tooth loss, sickly pallor, fatigue, partial paralysis, gout, depression, paranoia, mood swings, headaches, insomnia, fits, blindness, low sex drive, low fertility, and coma.

Mercury: a mineral in either liquid form, known as quicksilver, or an ore called mercury sulfide, another name for cinnabar, a red mineral from which quicksilver can be extracted.

Poisoning symptoms: excessive salivation; bad breath; inflamed lips, gums, and teeth; loss of teeth and gum tissue; kidney damage. Affects the central nervous system, causing tremors, shaking, and spidery handwriting. Causes mental deterioration, paranoia, mood swings, outbursts of anger, depression, poor concentration, and insomnia.

Ingesting quicksilver is oddly nontoxic as the substance generally passes through the gut unabsorbed, though ingesting it in the form of mercury sublimate is quite deadly. Mercury absorbed in any form through the skin is dangerous, and inhaled mercury is often fatal as the fumes cause significant brain damage.

PLANT POISONS

Aconite, also known as Monks-Hood or Wolf's Bane: a genus of over 250 species of flowering, perennial plants.

Poisoning symptoms: nausea, vomiting, diarrhea, a burning and numbness in the mouth and face that can spread to the limbs, sweating, dizziness, difficulty in breathing, headache, confusion, and paralysis of the heart and lungs leading to death.

Belladonna or Deadly Nightshade: a perennial herbaceous plant in the tomato family. Belladonna means "beautiful woman" in Italian because fashionable ladies put its juice into their eyes to dilate their pupils.

Poisoning symptoms: extreme dryness of the mouth and throat, loss of balance, scarlet rash, slurred speech, blurred vision, sensitivity to light, urinary retention, constipation, confusion, hallucinations, delirium, and convulsions.

Foxglove or Digitalis: a genus of about twenty species of herbaceous perennials, shrubs, and biennials with beautiful purple flowers.

Poisoning symptoms: confusion, irregular heartbeat, nausea, vomiting, diarrhea, distorted vision, difficulty breathing, and heart block.

Hellebore: comprises twenty species of herbaceous or evergreen perennial flowering plants.

Poisoning symptoms: tinnitus, vertigo, stupor, thirst, a feeling of suffocation, swelling of the tongue and throat, vomiting, slow heart rate, collapse and death from cardiac arrest.

Hemlock: a highly poisonous perennial herbaceous flowering plant in the carrot family.

Poisoning symptoms: dizziness and numbness in the legs that spread upward until the heart and lungs are paralyzed.

Henbane: a plant related to belladonna.

Poisoning symptoms: similar to those of belladonna with the added danger of causing victims to fall into a deep sleep from which they never wake.

Poisonous Mushrooms: usually have white gills, a warty cap, a hollow stem, milky juice, and often change color when cut or broken.

Poisoning symptoms: prostration, headache, stupor, wild delirium, bloody diarrhea, stomach pain, vomiting, liver and kidney damage, cardiac paralysis, coma, and death.

Opium: the juice of the unripe seed capsules of the poppy plant.

Poisoning symptoms: an intense itching of the nose, a deep sleep, and gradual paralysis of the heart and lungs resulting in death.

Yew: a conifer tree with red berries.

Poisoning symptoms: rapid heart rate, muscle tremors, convulsions, collapse, difficulty breathing, circulation impairment, and eventually cardiac arrest. Sometimes there are no symptoms at all, however, and a few hours after ingestion the victim simply hits the ground dead.

ANIMAL POISONS

Cantharides or Spanish Fly: an emerald green beetle common throughout Europe.

Poisoning symptoms: burns and blistering all through the digestive and urinary tracts, convulsions, kidney failure, organ failure, and death.

Snake, scorpion, and sting ray: toxins are rarely harmful when ingested.

POST-RENAISSANCE POISONS

Cyanide: a chemical compound discovered in 1782 by a Swedish chemist. Obtained from bitter almonds, the pits of plums, apricots, and cherries, and apple seeds.

Poisoning symptoms: similar to those of altitude sickness because it prevents the body's cells from using oxygen, which all cells need to survive. Weakness, confusion, strange behavior, excessive sleepiness, coma, shortness of breath, headache, dizziness, seizures, and death.

Polonium-210: a highly unstable, silvery radioactive metal discovered in uranium ore in 1898 by Marie and Pierre Curie and named after Marie's homeland, Poland; a million times more deadly than cyanide.

Poisoning symptoms: severe headaches, extreme vomiting, diarrhea, hair loss, liver and kidney damage. Within a day or two of exposure, the victim looks like he or she is at the end stage of cancer. Death occurs after a few days or weeks.

Ricin: a toxic protein discovered in the beanlike seeds of the castor-oil plant by a German scientist in 1888, one of the most toxic substances known.

Poisoning symptoms: inhaled ricin causes fever, cough, severe difficulty breathing, and fluid in the lungs. Ingested ricin causes intestinal bleeding and organ damage. Death usually occurs within three days. Even a small amount can be fatal.

Sarin: a nerve agent and chemical compound created in the early 1940s by Nazi scientists as a chemical weapon.

Poisoning symptoms: nausea, diarrhea, vomiting, seizures, muscle spasms, and difficulty breathing occur as the poison attacks the nervous system. Death will usually occur as a result of asphyxia.

Strychnine: discovered by French chemists in 1818 from the Saint-Ignatius's-bean.

Poisoning symptoms: causes the most painful and horrific symptoms of any known poison. Within ten or twenty minutes after exposure, the body's muscles begin to spasm, starting with the head and neck and spreading throughout the body, with nearly continuous convulsions. Death comes from asphyxiation or exhaustion from the convulsions within two to three hours after exposure.

TCCD: a chemical compound also known as dioxin, the general name for a family of chlorinated hydrocarbons. First created in the late nineteenth century as a by-product of the burning of organic materials.

Odorless and tasteless. An ingredient in Agent Orange, it is 170,000 times more poisonous than cyanide.

Poisoning symptoms: acute pancreatitis, severe upper abdominal pain, nausea, vomiting, fever, chills, rapid heartbeat, loss of appetite, shock, respiratory distress, chloracne (a jaundiced, bloated, pockmarked face), cancer, death.

VX: a man-made chemical compound, more potent than sarin, that poisons through inhalation or skin absorption. VX disrupts the nervous and muscular systems, causing paralysis of the diaphragm, resulting in death by asphyxiation.

Poisoning symptoms: Sweating and muscular twitching at the area of exposure, nausea, vomiting, difficulty breathing, death.

The POISON HALL of FAME

Most painful death: Strychnine, which causes the entire body to spasm in excruciating, violent convulsions until the victim dies from exhaustion or asphyxiation two to three hours after exposure.

Easiest death: Hemlock. Numbness spreads slowly from the legs upward until it paralyzes the heart and lungs. In 399 bc, the Greek philosopher Socrates, condemned to death by the Athenian government, drank a cup of hemlock surrounded by friends and spoke cheerfully until the moment before he died.

Fastest acting: Cyanide. Inhaling a high concentration causes a coma with seizures and cardiac arrest within minutes. A major component of Zyklon B, the gas used by the Nazis to exterminate Jews in concentration camps.

Most disgusting symptoms: Long-term mercury exposure. Horrific bad breath. Black teeth. Excessive, stinking black saliva that causes the victim to constantly spit. Loss of teeth, jawbone, tongue, palate, and gum tissue. Oozing sores on the throat, lungs, mouth, and inside the cheeks. Lifelong tremors, staggering, and convulsions.

The biggest stomach blaster: Arsenic, which causes hours of projectile vomiting and explosive diarrhea until the victim is so severely dehydrated he or she closely resembles a corn husk.

The worst poison for your complexion: TCCD, which within hours of exposure creates blackheads, cysts, pustules, tumors, bloating, and pockmarks in the face called chloracne.

Poisons that turn friends into enemies: Chronic lead and mercury poisoning causes violent mood swings, paranoia, insomnia, outbursts of anger, and depression. Mercury- and lead-based paints likely contributed to the mood swings of history's most temperamental artists.

The term "mad as a hatter" comes from hat makers who inhaled mercury fumes while turning fur into felt. Interestingly, the introduction of mercury to hat making was due to the spread of syphilis across Europe in the sixteenth century. Hat makers collected their own urine to remove the fur from animal skin, and those hat makers undergoing mercury cures for syphilis produced superior felt. Mercury, they realized, must be excreted in urine. Hat makers started adding mercury directly to the felt-making mixture.

BIBLIOGRAPHY

Allen, A. M. *A History of Verona*. New York: Putman, 1910.

Al-'Ubaydi, Mohammed. *Khattab (1969–2002)*. West Point, NY: Combatting Terrorism Center at West Point. No date.

Ball, Philip. *The Devil's Doctor: Paracelsus and the World of Renaissance Magic and Science*. New York: Farrar, Straus and Giroux, 2006.

Bevan, Bryan. *Charles II's Minette*. London: Ascent Books, 1979.

Boorde, Andrew. *Dyetary of Helth*. London: Robert Wyer, 1542.

Borman, Tracy. *The Private Lives of the Tudors: Uncovering the Secrets of Britain's Greatest Dynasty*. London: Hodder and Stoughton, 2016.

Bowsky, William M. *Henry VII in Italy*. Lincoln: University of Nebraska Press, 1960.

Brantôme, Seigneur de Pierre de Bourdeille. *Illustrious Dames of the Court of the Valois Kings*. New York: The Lamb Publishing Co., 1912.

Brown, Horatio F., ed. *Calendar of State Papers Relating to English Affairs*. Volume 12, *1610–1613*. London: Mackie & Co., 1905.

Cartwright, Julia. *Madame: A Life of Henrietta, Daughter of Charles I and Duchess of Orleans*. London: Seeley and Co., Ltd., 1894.

Casparsson, Ragnar, Gunnar Ekström, and Carl-Herman Hjortsjö. *Erik XIV, Gravöppningen 1958 I Västerås Domkyrka.* Stockholm: P.A. Norstedt & Söner, 1962.

Castiglione, Baldassare. *The Book of the Courtier.* New York: Charles Scribner's Sons, 1903.

Cellini, Benvenuto. *The Autobiography of Benvenuto Cellini.* New York: Penguin, 1956.

Chamberlin, E. R. *The Fall of the House of Borgia.* New York: Dorset Press, 1974.

Chaplin, Arnold. *The Illness and Death of Napoleon Bonaparte (A Medical Criticism).* London: Alexander Stenhouse, 1913.

Cornwallis, Sir Charles. *The life and death of our late most incomparable and heroique prince, Henry Prince of Wales.* London: John Dawson, 1641.

Cortese, Isabella. *The Secrets of Signora Isabella Cortese.* Venice: Giovanni Bariletto, 1561.

Crawfurd, Raymond, MD. *The Last Days of Charles II.* Oxford: Clarendon Press, 1909.

Cronin, Vincent. *Napoleon Bonaparte: An Intimate Biography.* New York: William Morrow, 1972.

Denton, C. S. *Absolute Power: The Real Lives of Europe's Most Infamous Rulers.* London: Eagle Editions, 2006.

Desclozeaux, Adrien. *Gabrielle d'Estrées.* London: Arthur Humphreys, 1907.

D'Orliac, Jehanne. *The Lady of Beauty, Agnes Sorel.* Philadelphia: J. B. Lippincott, 1931.

Downing, Sarah Jane. *Beauty and Cosmetics 1550–1950.* Oxford: Shire Publications, 2015.

Elyot, Sir Thomas. *The Castle of Health.* London: The Widow Orwin, 1539.

Emsley, John. *The Elements of Murder, A History of Poison.* Oxford: Oxford University Press, 2005.

Farmer, James Eugene. *Versailles and the Court under Louis XIV.* New York: The Century Company, 1905.

Ferri, Maro, and Donatella Lippi. *I Medici, La Dinastia dei Misteri.* Florence, Italy: Giunti Editore, 2007.

Fraser, Antonia. *Royal Charles: Charles II and the Restoration.* New York: Alfred A. Knopf, 1979.

Freer, Martha Walker. *Henri IV and Marie de Medici.* London: Hurst and Blackett, 1861.

Freer, Martha Walker. *Jeanne d'Albret, Queen of Navarre.* London: Hurst and Blackett, no date.

Funck-Brentano, Frantz. *Princes and Poisoners: Studies of the Court of Louis XIV.* London: Duckworth & Co., 1901.

Gilder, Joshua, and Anne-Lee Gilder. *Heavenly Intrigue: Johannes Kepler, Tycho Brahe, and the Murder Behind One of History's Greatest Scientific Discoveries.* New York: Anchor Books, 2005.

Graham-Dixon, Andrew. *Caravaggio: A Life Sacred and Profane.* New York: W. W. Norton, 2010.

Hibbert, Christopher. *George III: A Personal History.* London: Viking, 1998.

Hilton, Lisa. *Athénaïs, The Real Queen of France: The Life of Louis XIV's Mistress.* New York: Little, Brown, 2002.

Holmes, Frederick. *The Sickly Stuarts: The Medical Downfall of a Dynasty.* Sparkford, UK: J. H. Haynes, 2003.

Hutton, Ulrich von. *De Morbo Gallico: A Treatise on the French Disease.* London: John Clark, 1730.

La Fayette, Marie-Madeleine Pioche de La Vergne. *The Secret History of Henrietta, Princess of England, First Wife of Philippe, Duc d'Orléans.* New York: E. P. Dutton, 1929.

Levy, Joel. *Poison: An Illustrated History.* Guilford, CT: Lyons Press, 2011.

Lewis, Paul. *Lady of France: A Biography of Gabrielle d'Estrées, Mistress of Henry the Great.* New York: Funk & Wagnalls, 1963.

Macauley, Thomas. *The History of England from the Time of James II.* Philadelphia: Porter & Coates, 1848.

Mackowiak, Philip A., MD. *Diagnosing Giants: Solving the Medical Mysteries of Thirteen Patients Who Changed the World.* Oxford: Oxford University Press, 2013.

Mackowiak, Philip A., MD. *Post Mortem: Solving History's Great Medical Mysteries.* Philadelphia: American College of Physicians, 2007.

MacLeod, Catherine. *The Lost Prince: The Life & Death of Henry Stuart*. London: National Portrait Gallery, 2012.

Melograni, Piero. *Wolfgang Amadeus Mozart: A Biography*. Chicago: University of Chicago Press, 2007.

Moulton, Thomas. *This is the Myrour or Glasse of Helth Necessary and Nedefull for Every Person to Loke In, That Wyll Kepe Theyr Body from the Syckenes of the Pestylynce*. London: Hugh Jackson, 1580.

Nada, John. *Carlos the Bewitched: The Last Spanish Hapsburg*. London: Jonathan Cape, 1962.

Packard, Francis R. *Life and Times of Ambroise Paré*. New York: Paul B. Hoeber, 1921.

Paliotti, Guido. *La Morte d'Arrigo VII di Lussemburgo*. Montepulciano, Italy: Tipografia Unione Cooperative, 1894.

Paré, Ambroise. *The Workes of that famous Chirurgion Ambrose Parey, Translated out of Latine and compared with the French*. London: Richard Cotes and R. Young, 1649.

Payne, Francis Loring, *The Story of Versailles*. New York: Moffat, Yard, 1919.

Pemell, Robert. *A Treatise on the Diseases of Children; with their Causes, Signs, Prognosticks, and Cures, for the benefit of such as do not understand the Latine Tongue, and very useful for all such as are House-keepers and have Children*. London: J. Legatt, 1653.

Prescott, Orville. *Lords of Italy*. New York: Harper and Row, 1932.

Roberts, Michael. *The Early Vasas: A History of Sweden 1523–1611*. Cambridge: Cambridge University Press, 1968.

Roelker, Nancy Lyman. *Queen of Navarre: Jeanne d'Albret 1528–1572*. Cambridge, MA: Harvard University Press, 1968.

Ruscelli, Girolamo. *The Secrets of the Reverend Maister Alexis of Piemont, Containing Excellent Remedies Against Diverse Diseases, Wounds, and Other Accidents, with the Maner to Make Distillations, Parfumes, Confitures, Dyings, Colours, Fusions, and Meltings*. London: Thomas Wright, 1595.

Scully, Terence. *The Art of Cookery in the Middle Ages*. Berlin: Boye6, 2005.

Skidmore, Chris. *Edward VI: The Lost King of England.* New York: St. Martin's Press, 2007.

Somerset, Anne. *Ladies-in-Waiting from the Tudors to the Present Day.* London: Weidenfeld & Nicolson, 1984.

Somerset, Anne. *Unnatural Murder: Poison at the Court of James I.* London: Orion Books, 1997.

Spangenberg, Hans. *Cangrande della Scala.* Berlin: R. Gaertners Verlagsbuchhandlung, 1892.

Stanley, Arthur Penrhyn. *Historic Memorials of Westminster Abbey.* London: John Murray, 1886.

Steegmann, Mary G. *Bianca Cappello.* Baltimore: Norman, Remington, 1913.

Sugg, Richard. *Mummies, Cannibals and Vampires: The History of Corpse Medicine from the Renaissance to the Victorians.* Routledge: New York, 2011.

Sully, Maximilian de Bethune, duke of. *Memoirs of Maximilian de Bethune, Duke of Sully, Prime Minister to Henry the Great.* Edinburgh: A. Donaldson, 1770.

Tracey, Larissa, ed. *Medieval and Early Modern Murder.* Cambridge: D. S. Brewer, 2018.

Troyat, Henri. *Ivan the Terrible.* New York: Berkley Books, 1982.

Warner, the Reverend Richard. *Antiquitates Culinariae, or Curious Tracts Relating to the Culinary Affairs of the Old English.* London: Robert Blamire, 1791.

Weider, Ben, and David Hapgood. *The Murder of Napoleon.* New York: Congdon & Lattès, 1982.

Wheeler, Jo. *Renaissance Secrets: Recipes & Formulas.* London: V & A Publishing, 2009.

Whorton, James C. *The Arsenic Century: How Victorian Britain Was Poisoned at Home, Work & Play.* Oxford: Oxford University Press, 2010.

Williams, Robert C. *The Forensic Historian: Using Science to Reexamine the Past.* New York: M. E. Sharpe, 2013.

Woolly, Hannah. *The Accomplisht Ladys Delight in Preserving, Physick, Beautifying, and Cookery.* London: B. Harris, 1675.

Ziegler, Gilette. *At the Court of Versailles, Eyewitness Reports from the Reign of Louis XIV.* New York: Dutton, 1966.

ARTICLES

Apostoli, Pietro, et al. "Multielemental Analysis of Tissues from Cangrande della Scala, Prince of Verona, in the 14th Century." *Journal
of Analytical Toxicology* 33 (July/August 2009): 322–27.

Barker, Sheilah. "The Art of Poison: The Medici Archives." *The Florentine* 85 (2008).

Baron, Jeremy Hugh. "Paintress, Princess and Physician's Paramour:
Poison or Perforation?" *Journal of the Royal Society of Medicine* 91
(April 1998): 213–16.

Bloch, Harry, MD. "Poisons and Poisoning: Implication of Physicians
with Man and Nations." *Journal of the National Medical Associa-
tion* 79, no. 7 (July 1987): 761–64.

Charlier, Philippe. "Autopsie des Restes de Diane de Poitiers." *La Revue du Practicien* 60 (2010): 290–93.

Charlier, Philippe. "L'évolution des Procédures d'embaumement aristo-
cratique en France médiévale et moderne (Agnès Sorel, Le Duc de Berry,
Louis XI, Charlotte de Savoie, Louis XII, Louis XIV et Louis XVIII)."
Medicina Nei Secoli Arte e Scienza 18, no. 3 (2006): 777–98.

Charlier, Philippe. "Qui a tué la Dame de Beauté? Étude Scientifique
des restes d'Agnès Sorel (1422–1450)." *Histoire des Sciences Médi-
cales* 40, no. 3 (2006): 255–66.

Charlier, Philippe. "Vie et mort de la Dame de Beauté, l'étude médi-
cale des restes d'Agnès Sorel." *La Revue du Practicien* 55 (2005):
1734–37.

Charlier, Philippe, et al. "The Embalming of John of Lancaster, First
Duke of Bedford (1435 A.D.): A Forensic Analysis." *Medicine, Science and the Law* 56, no. 2 (2016): 107–15.

Charlier, Philippe, et al. "Fatal Alchemy. Did Gold Kill a 16th Century
French Courtesan and Favourite of Henri II?" *BMJ* (December 19–
26, 2009): 1402–3.

Cillier, L., and F. P. Retief. "Poisons, Poisoning and the Drug Trade in
Ancient Rome." *Akroterion* 45 (2000): 88–100.

Clark, Doug Bock. "The Untold Story of the Accidental Assassins of
North Korea." *GQ*, October 2017.

Colman, Eric, MD. "The First English Medical Journal: Medicina Cu-
riosa." *The Lancet* 354 (July 24, 1999): 324–26.

Cox, Timothy M., et al. "King George III and Porphyria: An Elemental Hypothesis and Investigation." *The Lancet* 366 (July 23, 2005): 332–35.

Cumston, Charles Green, MD. "The Medicolegal Aspect and Criminal Procedure in the Poison Cases of the Sixteenth Century." *American Medicine* 11, no. 2 (January 13, 1906).

Cumston, Charles Green, MD. "The Victims of the Medicis and the Borgias in France from a Medical Standpoint." *Albany Medical Annals* 27 (August 1906): 567–90.

Derbyshire, David. "Mercury Poisoned Ivan the Terrible's Mother and Wife." *The Telegraph*, March 14, 2001.

Fornaciari, Gino. "The Aragonese Mummies of the Basilica of Saint Domenico Maggiore in Naples." *Medicina nei Secoli* 18, no. 30 (2006): 843–64.

Fornaciari, Gino. "Identificazione di agenti patogeni in serie scheletriche antiche: l'esempio della malaria dei granduchi de' Medici (Firenze, XVI secolo)." *Medicina nei Secoli Arte e Scienza* 22, no. 1–3 (2010): 261–72.

Fornaciari, Gino. "Malaria Was the 'Killer' of Francesco I de' Medici (1531–1587)." *American Journal of Medicine* 123, no. 6 (June 2010): 568–69.

Fornaciari, Gino. "A Medieval Case of Digitalis Poisoning: The Sudden Death of Cangrande Della Scala, Lord of Verona (1291–1329)." *Journal of Archeological Science* 54 (2015): 162–67.

Fornaciari, Gino. "Plasmodium falciparum Immunodetection in Bone Remains of Members of the Renaissance Medici Family (Florence, Italy, Sixteenth Century)." *Transactions of the Royal Society of Tropical Medicine and Hygiene* 104 (2010): 583–87.

Fornaciari, G. "Riscontri Obiettivi sulle tecniche di imbalsamazione in età moderna nelle mummie dell'Italia centro-Meridionale." *Medicina ne Secoli Arte e Scienza*, Supplemento no. 1 (2005): 257–324.

Frith, John. "Arsenic—the 'Poison of Kings' and the 'Saviour of Syphilis.'" *Journal of Military and Veterans' Health* 21, no. 4 (2013).

Gedmin, Jeffrey. "A Short History of Russian Poisoning." *American Interest* (June 4, 2015).

Guiffra, Valentina, et al. "Embalming Methods and Plants in Renaissance

Italy: Two Artificial Mummies from Siena (Central Italy)." *Journal of Archeological Science* 38 (2011): 1949–56.

Holmes, Grace, MD, and Frederick Holmes, MD. "The Death of Young King Edward VI." *New England Journal of Medicine* 345, no. 1 (July 5, 2001).

Kennedy, Maev. "Questions Raised Over Queen's Ancestry after DNA Test on Richard III's Cousins." *The Guardian*, December 2, 2014.

Kramer, Andrew E. "More of Kremlin's Opponents Are Ending Up Dead." *New York Times*, August 20, 2016.

Lewis, Jack. "Lead Poisoning, A Historical Perspective." *EPA Journal* (May 1985).

Mari, Francesco, et al. "The Mysterious Death of Francesco I de' Medici and Bianca Cappello: An Arsenic Murder?" *BMJ* 333 (December 23–30, 2006): 1299–1301.

Moore, Norman, MD. "An Historical Case of Typhoid Fever." *St. Bartholomew's Hospital Reports* 17 (1881): 135–50.

Politskovskaya, Anna. "Poisoned by Putin." *The Guardian*, September 9, 2004.

Röhl, John. "The Royal Family's Toxic Time-Bomb." *University of Sussex Newsletter*, June 25, 1999.

Roland, Christell, and Bernt Sjöstrand. "A Simplified Method for the Determination of Arsenic by Means of Activation Analysis." *Acta Chemica Scandinavica* 16 (1952): 2123–30.

Saltini, G. E. "Della Morte di Francesco I de' Medici e di Bianca Cappello." *Archivio storico italiano, Nuova serie* 18 (1863): 21–81.

Samuel, Henry. "Vladimir Putin and His Poison Tasters: Culinary Secrets of the World's Leaders." *Telegraph*, July 24, 2012.

Spurrell, Rev. F. "Notes on the Death of King John." *Archeological Journal* 38, no. 1 (1881).

Travis, Alan. "Why the Princes in the Tower Are Staying Six Feet Under." *The Guardian*, February 5, 2013.

Vellev, Jens. "Tycho Brahes liv, død og efterliv." *25 Søforklaringer*, Arhus Universitatsverlage (January 2012): 349–65.

UNATTRIBUTED ARTICLES

"Enrico VII non venne ucciso. Mor curandosi con l'arsenico." *La Nazione*, December 30, 2016.

"How Important Is Lead Poisoning to Becoming a Legendary Artist?" *The Atlantic*, November 25, 2013.

"Murder Among Medicis." *Newsweek*, January 9, 2007.

"The Mystery of Caravaggio's Death Solved at Last—Painting Killed Him." *The Guardian*, June 16, 2010.

"Russian Agent's Autopsy Was 'One of the Most Dangerous . . . in the Western World." *Daily News*, January 28, 2015.

WEBSITE ARTICLES

Lindsay, Suzanne Glover. "The Revolutionary Exhumations at St-Denis, 1793." Essay in *Conversations: An Online Journal of the Center for the Study of Material and Visual Cultures of Religion* (2014). DOI:10.22332/con.ess.2015.2

Retief, Francois P., and Louise Cilliers. "Poisons, Poisoning and Poisoners in Rome." *Medicina Antiqua*, Wellcome Trust Centre for the History of Medicine. http://www.ucl.ac.uk/~ucgajpd/medicina%20antiqua/index.html

Thompson, Helen. "Poison Hath Been This Italian Mummy's Untimely End." Smithsonian.com, April 10, 2016. http://www.smithsonianmag.com/science-nature/poison-hath-been-italian-mummys-untimely-end-digitalis-foxglove-180953822

Woollaston, Victoria. "Autopsy on 700-Year-Old Mummy Solves 14th Century Murder Mystery—Italian Lord Was Poisoned." DailyMail.com, April 10, 2016. http://www.dailymail.co.uk/sciencetech/article-2900693/Mystery-Cangrande-s-mummy-solved-Autopsy-tests-reveal-Lord-Verona-POISONED-foxglove-14th-century.html

UNATTRIBUTED WEBSITE ARTICLES

"King George III: Mad or Misunderstood?" BBCNews.com, July 13, 2004. http://news.bbc.co.uk/2/hi/health/3889903.stm

"Tsaritsas' Hair Solves the Mystery of Their Death." Freerepublic.com, July 29, 2002. http://www.freerepublic.com/focus/news/724240/posts

"Who Ordered Khattab's Death?" *North Caucasus Analysis* 3, no. 15 (May 29, 2002).

INDEX

Abbott, George, 184
Accomplisht Ladys Delight, 38
aconite, description, 262–263
Adams, Thomas, 15
Agent Orange, 249, 266
Agrippa, Cornelius, 47
Alexander the Great, 60, 222
Allbutt, Thomas, 234
animal poisons
    description, 264
anthrax, 86, 88–89, 219, 236
antimony, 3, 36, 38, 43, 50, 53, 60, 77, 78
    description, 261
Antoinette, Marie, 67
Arafat, Yasser, 254–256
arsenic
    accidental poisoning by, 12
    antidotes/protection from, 23–24
    Cangrande's poisoning, 93–94
    chemical studies of, 77–78, 234
    in clothing and decor, 240–241
    cosmetics and, 32–33, 36
    description, 261-262
    Eric XIV's poisoning, 123, 127–128
    Francesco I de Medici's poisoning,
        142–145
    hair and, 41

Henrietta Stuart's poisoning, 201
Ivan the Terrible and, 135–136
medicine and, 43, 48, 50, 53, 89,
    239–240
Napoleon and, 229–230
paint and, 171
porphyria and, 59–60
Renaissance poisoning and, 3–5
symptoms of poisoning, 14–15
tests for, 239
Thomas Overbury's poisoning,
    187–188
treatment of lice, 39–40
Tycho Brahe's poisoning, 161
vomiting to avoid poisoning by, 26
Audley, Thomas, 106
availability of poisons
    clothing, chemicals in, 240–241
    home goods, chemicals in, 240
    wallpaper, chemicals in, 240

Bacon, Sir Francis, 192
Baer, Nicholas Reimers, 159
Baglione, Giovanni, 167
Barclay, David, 255
belladonna, 5, 36
    description, 263

bezoar stones, 22, 29–30, 37, 76,
        141, 178
Black Death, 72. *See also plague*
bloodletting, 43, 45
Bodle, John, 234–235
Bonaparte, Napoleon, xii, 83–84, 221–230,
        233, 240
    battles, 224–226
    contemporary postmortem, 228–229
    illness and death, 228
    imprisonment at St. Helena, 226–228
    modern diagnosis, 229–230
    rule of France, 223–224
Borgia family. *See also Pope Alexander VI*
    Cesare, 12, 15
    Rodrigo, 12
Boscher, Alexander, 200–201
Brahe, Tycho
    advances in astronomy, 156–158
    background, 155–156
    Kepler, Johannes and, 158–159
    modern postmortem and diagnosis,
        161–163
    poisoning and death, 159–161
Bullein, William, 36
Burbury, John, 66

Calvin, John, 117–118
Cangrande della Scala
    background, 91–92
    modern postmortem and diagnosis,
        93–95
    poisoning and death, 92–93
cantharides / Spanish fly, 76, 187–188
    description, 264
Caravaggio (Michaelangelo Merisi),
        165–172
    background, 165–167
    duel with Ranuccio da Terni, 168
    induction to Knights of Malta, 168
    injuries and death, 169–170
    postmortem and diagnosis, 170–172
    works, 167–168
Caravita, Gregorio, 28
Carr, Anne, 192
Carr, Robert, 179, 184, 189–192
Castiglione, Baldassare, 32
Cecil, William, 11

Cellini, Benvenuto, 20
Chapelain, Jean, 21
chelation, 23
cholera, 73, 200–201
civil wars
    English, 106, 181, 192–193
    French, 118, 147, 149
    Italian, 84
clothing, chemicals in, 240–241
Colbert, Charles, 197
Columbus, Christopher, 50
Cornwallis, Charles, 176
Cortile, Ercole, 27
cosmetics
    aqua argentata, 37–38
    arsenic face powder, 33
    beauty and, 31–32
    belladonna, 36
    Diane de Poitiers and, 40–42
    Elizabeth I and, 31–34
    hair and wigs, 38–39
    heavy metal poisoning, 33
    lead and, 32–33
    lice and, 39–40
    mercury-based, 33, 37
    ox dung, 38
    sin and, 32
    smallpox scars and, 32
    soaking in blood, 35–36
    urine, 36–37
Cotesworth, William, 69
Council of Ten, 4, 28
Croll, Oswald, 56
Culpeper, Nicholas, 47
cyanide, 244–245, 249, 251, 256,
        266–267
    description, 264

d'Aragona, Isabella, 54–55
d'Aubigné, Agrippa, 151
d'Estrées, Gabrielle
    background, 147–151
    contemporary postmortem, 152–153
    modern diagnosis, 153
    poisoning and death, 151–152
Dante Alighieri, 85, 92
de Coligny, Gaspard II, 121
de Coligny, Odet, 16

de Luca, Tolomeo, 87
de Mayerne, Théodore, 55
de Montepulciano, Bernadino, 87
De Morbo Gallicus (de Vigo), 52
de Quevedo, Francisco, 62
de Vigo, Giovanni, 52
dead birds, 49, 177
deadly nightshade. *See* belladonna
Defoe, Daniel, 74
del Monte, Francesco Maria Bourbon, 167
della Casa, Giovanni, 68
Devereux, Robert, Earl of Essex, 12, 183
diamonds, as protection against poison, 22, 45
Diaz, Ruy, 50
Disraeli, Benjamin, 73
Doan Thi Huong, 257
Duchess Bianca Capello
    background, 137–138
    children, 139–140
    contemporary postmortems, 142–143
    marriage to Duke Francesco I de Medici, 138–139
    modern postmortem and dueling diagnoses, 143–146
    poisoning and death, 140–142
Dudley, John (Earl of Warwick), 107
Duke Cosimo I, 3–4, 26–28, 138
dung, medical uses of
    mice, 48
    ox, 38, 48
    rooster, 26

E. coli, 14
Elyot, Thomas, 44
Emperor Francis II (Austria), 224–225
Emperor Henry VII (Luxembourg)
    anthrax and, 86–87
    background, 83–84
    death, 87–88
    Guelph Republic of Florence and, 85–86
    modern postmortem and diagnosis, 88–89
Emperor Joseph II, 215–217, 220

Emperor Nicholas II (Russia), 244
Evelyn, John, 67–68

Felix, Charles-François, 67
fistulas, 67
food poisoning, 14
food tasters, 6–8, 10, 19, 87, 102, 145
Fornaciari, Gino, 143
Forshufvud, Sten, 229
Fowler's Solution, 239
foxglove / digitalis, 14, 94
    description, 263
Fracastoro, Girolamo, 50
Frobisher, Martin, 20

gallows guinea pigs, 28–30
gallstones, 22. *See also bezoar stones*
gemstones, as protection from poison, 21–22, 26
Goya, Francisco, 171
Great Fire of 1547 (Russia), 131
Great Stink of 1858, 73
Grey, Jane, 109, 113, 190
Guelph Republic of Florence, 84–85, 87, 91

Harington, John, 33–34, 174
Harvey, William, 45, 234
Hastings, Henry (Earl of Huntington), 69
Hayward, John, 45
hellebore, 39
    description, 263
Helmont, Jean Baptiste van, 56
hemlock, 267
    description, 263
henbane, description, 263
Henrietta Stuart (Duchesse d'Orléans)
    background, 193–194
    contemporary postmortem, 200–201
    illness and death, 196–200
    modern diagnosis, 201–202
    public love for, 194–196
Henry Stuart (Prince of Wales), 173–181, 184, 188
    contemporary postmortem, 180
    illness, 175–180
    modern diagnosis, 181
    overview, 173–175
    Walter Raleigh and, 174, 178–179

Henry the Navigator (Prince), 157
Henry, Walter, 225
Hippocrates, 43
Hodgepodge of Various Secrets
    (Rosselli), 27
humors, 46–49, 52, 58, 67, 71, 76, 173,
    175–178, 183, 188, 236, 262
Hundred Years' War, 98
Hutten, Ulrich von, 51–52

industrialization, 239
Ivan the Terrible
    background, 129–132
    death of wife Anastasia, 132
    modern postmortems and diagnoses,
        135–136
    murder of son, 134
    poisoning and death, 134–135
    proposal to Elizabeth I, 133–134
    wives, 133

James's Powder, 60
Jeanne d'Albret (Queen of Navarre)
    background, 115–119
    contemporary postmortem, 120–121
    illness and death, 119–120
    modern diagnosis, 121–122
Joan of Arc, 98
John of Gaunt, 111
John of Lancaster, 135

Kara-Murza, Vladimir, 253–254
Khattab, Emir, 247–248
Kim Jong-nam, 256–258
Kim Jong-un, 256, 258
King Charles I (England), 111, 179–181,
    193–194, 196
King Charles II (England), 49, 55–56, 63,
    68–69, 75–78, 110, 196, 200
King Charles IX (France), 20, 29, 121,
    150
King Charles V (Spain), 22
King Charles VI (France), 98
King Charles VII (France), 70, 97, 103.
    See also Sorel, Agnes
King Charles VIII (France), 50
King Christian IV (Denmark), 55, 158,
    160, 178

King Christian V (Denmark), 20
King Edward VI (England), 7, 57, 63,
    105–113, 174
    background, 105–107
    contemporary postmortem, 110
    illness and death, 107–110
    modern diagnosis, 112–113
    poisoning, 109–110
    unlikelihood of a modern postmortem,
        110–112
King Erik XIV (Sweden)
    background, 123–126
    modern postmortem and diagnosis,
        127–128
    poisoning and death, 126–127
King François (France), 22
King George I (England), 64
King George III (England), 58–60, 239
King Henry IV (England), 69, 111
King Henry VII (England), 110, 112–113
King Henry VIII (England), 5, 7, 11, 31,
    46, 57, 61–63, 72, 105–106,
    108–109, 134, 150. *See also King
    Edward VI*
King James I (England), 35, 55, 59, 66,
    112, 173–177, 179, 183–187,
    190–191
King James VI (Scotland), 27
King Louis XI (France), 98–100
King Louis XIV (France), 9, 13, 63–64,
    66–67, 69–70, 74, 194–196,
    199–203, 205, 207, 209, 248, xi
King Louis XVI (France), 74
King Louis XVIII (France), 221–222, 225
King Robert of Naples, 85, 87
King Sigismund I (Poland), 20
King William II (England), 55
Koch, Robert, 58, 73, 113, 236
Koltsov, Nikolai Konstantinovich,
    244–245

Laënnec, René Theophile Hyacinthe, 233
Laird's Bloom of Youth, 239. *See also
    cosmetics*
Laveran, Charles Louis Alphonse, 236
lead, 3, 5, 24
    alchemy and, 75, 77
    coffins, 35, 40, 100–101

in cosmetics, 32–33, 36–37, 39,
    41
description, 262
effects of poisoning, 262, 268
in medicine, 43, 48, 52–53
Leared, Arthur, 234
leeches, 58. *See also bloodletting*
Leewenhoek, Anthony van, 235–236
Lenin, Vladimir, 245
Leonardus, Camillus, 22
lice, 39, 45, 48, 54–55, 68–70, 72, 135,
    230, xii
Life and Raigne of King Edward VI
    (Hayward), 45
Luddett, Edward, 75

Madame de Montespan, 204–211
Mademoiselle de Fontanges
    background, 203–207
    contemporary postmortem, 210
    Madame de Montespan and, 207–209
    modern diagnosis, 210–211
    poisoning and death, 203, 209–210
Magnitsky Act, 253
Maimonides, 5–7, 22, 26
Maister Alexis of Piedmont, 24–25,
    36–39, 42, 48
malaria, 14–15, 88, 101, 142–145, 165,
    170–171, 236
Mandeville, John, 22
Marchand, Louis, 228
Marie Antoniette, 67
Marsh test, 235, 241
Marsh, James, 234, 241
Mary, Queen of Scots, 59, 125, 193
Mattioli, Pietro Andrea, 28
Mayerne, Théodore de, 55, 59, 175–177,
    180, 188
Mayne, Michael, 110
Medici family, 26–28, 33, 71, 143,
    145–146, 152, 244
    Catherine de Medici, 16, 49, 57, 115,
        119, 150
    Duke Cosimo I, 3–4, 26–28, 138
    Ferdinando de Medici, 152, 183
    Francesco I de Medici, 137–146, 150,
        152, 167
    Marie de Medici, 150, 152

medicine
    apothecaries, 47
    astrology and, 45–46
    bloodletting, 45
    cannibal cures, 55–60
    dead birds, 49
    discovery of infectious disease, 58
    effects of poisonous medication, 58–59
    foods and, 44–45
    human blood and, 57
    human brain and, 56–57
    humors and, 43–44
    illness as, 45
    laxatives, 49–50
    lice and, 45
    lung ailments, 48–49
    mercury-based, 49, 52–55
    near-religious approach to, 46–47
    Paracelsus on, 46, 48
    porphyria and, 59–60
    puerperal fever, 57–58
    sexually-transmitted diseases, 50–55
    skin ailments, 48
mercury
    Agnes Sorel's poisoning, 98, 102, 183
    alchemy and, 75–76, 239–240, 259, 260
    antidotes/protection, 23–24
    chelation and, 23
    clays and, 24
    in cosmetics, 33, 37, 39, 41, 240
    described, 262
    Ivan the Terrible and, 135–136
    long-term exposure to, 267
    in medicine, 43, 48–50, 52–55, 89,
        259–260
    mood swings, 268
    paint and, 171
    Paré's study of, 25–26
    Renaissance-era poison and, 3–4, 13,
        18
    syphilis treatment, 52–55, 239
    Thomas Overbury's poisoning, 183,
        187–188
    Tycho Brahe's poisoning, 161–162
mice dung, 48
Mirror of Precious Stones, The
    (Leonardus), 22
Mithridates VI (King of Pontus), 23

modern cases of poisoning
  Arafat, Yasser, 254–256
  Kara-Murza, Vladimir, 253–254
  Kattab, Emir, 247–248
  Kim Jong-nam, 256–258
  Lenin, Vladimir and, 245–246
  Litvinenko, Alexander, 250–252
  Perepilichny, Alexander, 252–253
  Politkovskaya, Anna, 249–250
  Putin, Vladimir and, 243, 246
  Russian/Soviet political assassinations,
    243–247
  Sobchak, Anatoly and, 246–247
  Stalin, Joseph and, 245–246
  Yushchenko, Victor, 248–249
Montecuccoli, Sebastiano, 15
mortality rates, 51, 57–58, 86, 241
Moulton, Thomas, 45–46
Mozart, Leopold, 213–217
Mozart, Wolfgang Amadeus, 73, 213,
    215–220, ix, xii
  illness and death, 217–219
  modern diagnosis, 219–220
  overview, 213–216
  relationship with father, 214–216
  Salieri, Antonio and, 216–217
mushrooms, poisonous, 14, 23
  description, 263–264
Mussato, Albertino, 87–88

Napoleonic Wars, 233
Nashe, Thomas, 15
Neville, George, 8
Newton, Isaac, 77–78, 161
Northern Seven Years' War, 124
Northumberland, Duke, 107–109, 113

Oakes, Thomas, 75
Obama, Barack, 253
Oldenburg, Henry, 235
On the Motion of the Heart and Blood
    (Harvey), 234
opium, 23, 127
  description, 264
Overbury, Thomas, 14, 67, 183–192
  overview, 183–187
  poisoning and death, 187–192
ox dung, 38, 48

Paracelsus, 46–48, 55
Paré, Ambroise, 21
Pemell, Robert, 39, 45
Pinzón, Martin Alonso, 50
Pitt, Robert, 56
plague, 24, 27, 39, 46, 56, 72–74, 86,
    180, 236
poison detection/blocking
  diamonds, 22
  food tasters, 19
  gallows guinea pigs, 28–30
  gemstones, 21–22
  merits of vomiting, 24–28
  mithridate/theriac potions, 23–24
  toadstones, 22–23
  unicorn horns, 19–21
Poitevin, Robert, 102
polonium-210, 251, 254–256
  description, 264
Pope Alexander VI, 12–13, 15, 247
Pope Clement II, 171
Pope Clement V, 87
Pope Clement VII, 20, 28
Pope Leo X, 13–14
porphyria, 59–60, 229
Ptolemy, 156–157
puerperal fever, 57–58
Putin, Vladimir, 243, 246–253

Queen Anne (England), 174, 178–179
Queen Catherine (France), 119, 121
Queen Elizabeth I (England), 12, 20, 22,
    31, 33, 35, 38, 55, 66, 113, 174
Queen Elizabeth II, 59, 110–111
Queen Isabella (Spain), 50, 66
Queen Jane (England), 106
Queen Jeanne (France), 115, 149
Queen Marguerite of Navarre, 12
Queen Marie (France), 99
Queen Mary (England), 73
Queen Victoria (England), 59

Raleigh, Walter, 174
rat poison, 239
ricin, 246
  description, 265
rooster dung, 26
Ross, Ronald, 237

Rosselli, Stefano, 27–28
Russell, William (Duke of Bedford), 192

Saint-John's-wort, 23
Salieri, Antonio, 213, 216, 218–219
Salvarsan, 239
sanitation
    alchemy and, 75–78
    health risks of bathing, 65–68
    human waste, 61–65
    lice and fleas, 68–72
    toxic towns, 72–75
Santorio, Santorio, 234
sarin, 247
    description, 265
Scaramelli, Giovanni, 34
Scheele, Karl, 240
scientific advances
    blood circulation, 234
    chemistry, 234–235
    debunking of outdated practices,
        236–237
    measuring fevers, 254
    medical equipment, 233–234
    microscope, 235–236
Second Chechen War, 247
Secrets of Signora Isabella Cortese, 38
Semmelweis, Ignaz, 57–58
Seymour, Thomas, 57
Sforza, Francesco (Duke of Milan), 28
Shchekochikhin, Yuri Petrovich, 248
Siti Aisyah, 257
smallpox, 31–32, 45, 71, 73, 107, 158,
    180, 213
snake venom, 24
Snow, John, 73
Sobchak, Anatoly, 246
Socrates, 267
Sorel, Agnes
    background, 97–98
    beauty, 98–100
    modern postmortem and diagnosis,
        100–103
    relationship with Charles VI, 98–99
    relationship with Prince Louis,
        99–100
Squire, Edward, 12
Stalin, Joseph, 245–246

stethoscopes, 233–234
Strozzi, Piero, 3–4
strychnine, 252, 256, 267
    description, 265
syphilis
    Caravaggio, Michelangelo Merisi and,
        170
    Franklin, James and, 187
    history, 50–52
    Ivan the Terrible and, 136
    treatments for, 52–54, 239, 268
    Vincenti, Silvano and, 170

TCCD, 249, 268
    description, 265–266
terra sigilata, 24, 26, 29
This is the Myrour of Glasse of Helth
    (Moulton), 45
Throckmorton, John, 192
toadstones, 22
Treponema pallidum, 52, 54
trichinosis, 14
Tudors, 9, 64, 69, 190. See also King
    Edward VI; Queen Elizabeth I
typhoid, 73–74, 181

unicorn horns, 19–21, 26, 29, 129, 134,
    243
    debunking of healing properties, 21
    poison detection, 19–20
    reality of, 19
    value of, 20–21

van Diemerbroeck, Ysbrand, 71
Vibrio cholerae, 73. See also cholera
Villiers, George, 190–191
Virchow, Rudolph, 236
vitamin D defiency, 33, 71
Volodarsky, Boris, 244
vomiting, merits of, 24–28
VX, 256–257
    description, 266

Wade, William, 186
Walker, George "Graveyard," 74
wallpaper, chemicals in, 240
William of Gloucester, Prince, 59
Willis, Thomas, 48

Yersin, André, 236
Yersinia pestis, 72, 236
yew, 23
    description, 264
Yolande of Aragon, 98–99

Yushchenko, Viktor, 248–249. *See also
    modern cases of poisoning*

zodiac signs, 21, 44
Zyklon B, 267